Healing Depression & Bipolar D**Drugs**

Healing Depression & Bipolar Disorder Without Drugs

Inspiring Stories of Restoring Mental Health Through Natural Therapies

GRACELYN GUYOL

Walker & Company
NEW YORK

Published by Walker Publishing Company, Inc., New York
Distributed to the trade by Holtzbrinck Publishers.

All papers used by Walker & Company are natural, recyclable products made from wood grown in well-managed forests. The manufacturing processes conform to the environmental regulations of the country of origin.

Library of Congress Cataloging-in-Publication Data

Guyol, Gracelyn.
   Healing depression & bipolar disorder without drugs : inspiring stories of restoring mental health through natural therapies / Gracelyn Guyol.
      p. cm.
   Includes bibliographical references and index.
ISBN-13: 978-0-8027-1496-1 (pbk.)
ISBN-10: 0-8027-1496-X (pbk.)
   1. Depression, Mental.   2. Depression, Mental—Alternative treatment.
3. Manic depressive illness—Alternative treatment.   I. Title: Healing depression and bipolar disorder without drugs.   II. Title.
   RC537.G89 2006
   616.85'2706—dc22

                                                                    2005035506

Visit Walker & Company's Web site at www.walkerbooks.com

First U.S. edition 2006

2   4   6   8   10   9   7   5   3   1

Typeset by Westchester Book Group
Printed in the United States of America by Quebecor World Fairfield

*To my husband, Jack, for his love and support
through my difficult bipolar years*

and

*To Beth Walker, a founder of Walker Publishing,
for making this book a reality*

A Note from the Author

Do not discontinue or reduce your dose of psychiatric medications without the supervision of a physician. Your brain has adjusted to the drugs you are taking, and any sudden changes may cause serious reactions and endanger your health.

The ideas, processes, and suggestions contained in this book are not intended to replace the services of a trained health professional. Ask your doctor to help you find alternatives to prescription drugs. If your practitioner is not receptive to this approach, find a new one (see chapter 14 and resources) who understands alternative medical treatments and will work with you to eliminate the symptoms of depression or bipolar disorder. While this book is intended to provide information on new healing options, any application of the information is the reader's responsibility and must be undertaken only under the supervision of a trained health professional.

Accounts of healing in these chapters are based on real people and their experiences. Those identified by full names have chosen to become public advocates of natural therapies for mental health. Others who prefer privacy are identified by a single pseudonym.

Throughout the book I name many other books, products, companies, and practitioners. I do so as a service to readers. I receive no compensation nor do I have financial ties to any of them.

—*Gracelyn Guyol*

Contents

FOREWORD   Stephen T. Sinatra, M.D., F.A.C.C.   XI

INTRODUCTION   Why Drugs Are Not the Best Solution for
Mental Disorders   1

PART I   *Clearing Potential Underlying Biological Causes*

  1. Identifying and Compensating for Genetic Traits   27
  2. Brain Basics: Vitamins, Minerals, and Good Fats   44
  3. Ruling Out Hormone Imbalances, Diseases,
and Medications   60
  4. Rebuilding with Glyconutrients, Proteins, and
Amino Acids   77
  5. Hidden Triggers: Allergies, Food Sensitivities, and
Flawed Digestion   90
  6. Detoxification: Mercury, Pesticides, and
Other Poisons   106
  7. Halting *Candida albicans* (Yeast) Overgrowth   122
  8. Eliminating Parasite Infestations   136

PART II   *The Most Effective Nondrug Therapies*

  9. Neurofeedback: Retraining Brain Waves   149
 10. Releasing Trauma by Eye Movement
Desensitization & Reprocessing or Emotional
Transformation Therapy   158

11. Reconnecting Mind and Body: Prayer, Affirmations, Imagery, Yoga, and Meditation   170

12. Energy Healing: Therapeutic Touch, Reiki, and Acupuncture   184

13. Homeopathy: A Potent Medical System   196

PART III *Creating Your Future*

14. Restoring Mental Health   207

APPENDICES

APPENDIX A   Anti-Inflammatory Diet   223

APPENDIX B   Sample Candida Control Program by Infinity Health   227

APPENDIX C   Sample Antiprotozoa Program by Infinity Health   233

RESOURCES: Natural Alternatives for Healing   239

RECOMMENDED READING   247

NOTES   249

INDEX   271

Foreword

My initial interest in reading *Healing Depression & Bipolar Disorder Without Drugs* stemmed from my hope that perhaps we are beginning to identify the underpinnings of these two disorders, for only then can we begin to reduce the human suffering that they cause. Anyone who has been diagnosed with depression or bipolar disorder (BPD), or lives with someone who has, knows how seriously these conditions can blunt one's experience of the richness life has to offer.

You see, these maladies have impacted my own life on a very personal level. I grew up with two close family members who had BPD—my father and my maternal aunt—and I know the heartaches for both the afflicted and all who love and live with them. It's nothing less than a roller-coaster ride at times, and naturally my siblings and I worried that we might someday develop the same problems.

For my younger sister, who developed SAD, or seasonal affective disorder, her "cure"—a geographical move from northern Michigan and its long dark winters down to sunny Florida—was a better treatment than any medication. Light therapy was all she needed to totally eliminate her symptoms, and I am sure that similar nondrug solutions are realistic interventions for many others with less intense symptoms of anxiety or depression.

But can less toxic approaches be used to treat more serious and sometimes life-threatening cases of depression and BPD? I certainly would hope so, although such approaches should be pursued only under the close care of a trained professional who guides and evaluates the patient effectively. If you were to ask me whether I think that my dad's BPD was handled well by his traditionally trained physicians and the heavy-duty drugs he took, I would respond with a definite "No." Some of his symptoms were secondary to the side effects of the very medications that were used to keep him stabilized. There was even an occasion when I'm convinced his confused state was the result of a lithium toxicity combined with a blood-pressure-drug interaction. But his physicians wouldn't hear me, even though by then I was an M.D. myself.

Yet I also know my dad could have harmed himself or someone else when he became so manic that he was no longer the man I knew and loved so much. Then I realize that I was thankful for those same pharmaceutical interventions. That is the strained juxtaposition that we still face in medicine when treating any physical illness, be it primarily physical or mental.

So, the opportunity to read a book about new perspectives on healing people like my beloved father and my dear aunt was an opportunity I couldn't resist. And what an enjoyable read *Healing Depression & Bipolar Disorder Without Drugs* is. Gracelyn Guyol looks at more than treating the symptoms of these debilitating problems; her mission is to help you unearth some of the underlying causes so that you might begin a process of healing. But allow me to tell you a little of my own journey and the professional reasons why I find this book worthwhile.

I've practiced for over twenty years as an invasive cardiologist, which means that I perform procedures such as installing cardiac catheters, temporary pacemakers, and arterial lines as well as treating patients in the hospital and my office. But invasive cardiology wasn't enough to answer a lot of the questions I had about who has a heart attack, and why, and when.

Then, in the late 1970s, the idea that stress was connected to heart diseases found its way into the minds of the public long before it was ever accepted by the American Heart Association and most mainstream cardiologists. But I embraced the new research identifying Type A behavior and other ideas wholeheartedly. My search for answers led me into ten years of mind-body training in Gestalt and bioenergetic therapies, and certification in the latter. At last, I could feel completely comfortable running stress and illness seminars for cardiac patients. Finally, I had more to offer than pills and punctures, and my professional life took on more meaning for me.

Over the last twenty years, I have expanded my treatment modalities into the arena of "alternative" medicine. After much review of the research into the antioxidant craze of the mid-1980s, I became convinced that taking specific supplements and herbal remedies might be beneficial to the heart and body. It wasn't long before I found that I could no longer practice cardiology without targeted supplements, including nutrients and minerals like coenzyme Q10, magnesium, and L-carnitine, to mention a few. Everything changed for me in how I treated stable cardiology patients for hypertension, heart attack and heart surgery recovery, arrhythmias, and so on.

Now, I am committed to teaching physicians and the public how to care for their hearts and bodies with less toxic pharmaceutical approaches that don't involve side effects. I also address environmental toxicities and how they impact our cardiac and general health.

Therefore, when Gracelyn Guyol told me of her study into the use of supplements and other natural remedies in treating depression and bipolar disorder, I was intrigued and open-minded. I know of some "natural" approaches to anxiety and depression that helped my cardiac population, but I'm inexperienced in using them for more complex mental illnesses, such as overt mania or profound depression. I found *Healing Depression & Bipolar Disorder Without Drugs* insightful and right up my alley, so to speak. This book presents patients who have these two major psychiatric problems (and their families) with information about possible new contributing factors. In doing so, the book promotes the proactive approach that I always encourage in all my patients.

Often we view heart disease and mental illnesses as being based in genetics, which makes all of us feel like victims of our own particular fate, instead of active agents in our own recovery. While family history may make us vulnerable to particular medical conditions (I myself have a one-in-seven chance of developing bipolar disorder), environmental factors can trigger or aggravate one's predisposition. Gracelyn Guyol points out specific environmental issues that may be involved in these mental illnesses so that people can be tested for them and take action to address them. Read her book carefully, and see if you recognize any factors such as a toxic exposure or a nutritional deficiency that may be blocking your healing.

This may be the first time some of you consider both physical and mental health from the point of view of contamination and detoxification. But it is no secret that we do live in a toxic environment, and that the sea of chemicals permeating our air, water, and food will help to create not only physical illnesses such as heart disease and autoimmune disorders, but mental illness as well. Heavy metals, insecticides, pesticides, radiation, inflammation-provoking foods, dyes, and chemicals bombard us on a day-to-day basis. They create not only physical symptoms, but psychological and mental symptoms as well. Consider one such chemical: perchlorate, a former rocket fuel. It now has been found in the water supply of the southwestern United States, particularly in the Colorado River Basin. Perchlorate can be a source of profound thyroid dysfunction and cause overwhelming fatigue and depression.

Healing Depression & Bipolar Disorder Without Drugs reveals several ways a toxic environment can contaminate the body and cause illness. Certainly, we see many cases of chronic fatigue syndrome and fibromyalgia that are caused by exposure to toxic agents. Newer biotoxins, neurotoxins, and molds have also been recently discovered to cause other strange and debilitating illnesses. So can many biochemical conditions like bipolar disorder be initiated or exacerbated by exposure to toxic chemicals. And these environmental problems are literally causing intense pain and suffering, both physical and mental, for millions of people.

As a cardiologist, I understand how faulty metabolism of adenosine triphosphate, or ATP, causes all kinds of problems, from cardiac conditions to autoimmune disorders such as chronic fatigue syndrome and fibromyalgia. But developing more drugs to treat these maladies is not always the answer. I'm seeing more and more instances in my own practice where nutraceutical supports best help to correct some of these chemical-based problems. The trick in practicing medicine—and in making recommendations to the public—is finding the balance between traditional medical approaches and more natural solutions, whether it's taking supplements or having a chiropractic session and massage. So, my caveat to you when you read this book is that you keep in mind that medication intervention and natural approaches are not mutually exclusive.

Even though I choose to use interventions that treat cardiac patients in natural biochemical ways, I still have to use drug and surgical approaches in many situations, especially acute-care medicine. I could never treat an acute heart attack successfully without drugs such as nitroglycerine to relax blood vessels, streptokinase to dissolve clots, lidocaine to treat life-threatening arrhythmias, or angioplasty or bypass surgery in extreme cases.

Similarly, psychiatric emergencies may require drug interventions. Offering GABA or Saint-John's-wort (which you'll read about in this book) to someone having a major manic or depressive episode is like offering a vitamin E or coenzyme Q10 capsule to a patient having a major heart attack. Let me tell you about the first true psychiatric emergency I had to treat—so you understand why I caution everyone about relying solely on a natural approach to treat BPD.

During the winter of 1972, when I was a psychiatric resident on call at Albany Medical Center Hospital, I had to deal with many psychiatric emergencies. One evening when the emergency room was particularly overwhelmed with multiple trauma cases, a woman with BPD (I'll call her Mary) was brought in by her distressed family. Mary's daughter had called ahead and was advised to bring her mother at once. Mary arrived in full-blown mania, screaming at the top of her lungs, "Where's that Dr. Sinatra, that rotten S.O.B.??!!"

For any of you clinicians, family members, or friends who know some of the symptoms of an acute manic episode, you know that aggression, combativeness, impulsivity, impaired judgment, inappropriate behavior, psychotic thinking, and hypersexuality are just a few of the hallmarks. The ER nurses and staff tried their best to calm and reassure her, but Mary's outbursts could not be controlled. Her agitation only heightened with anything she perceived as confrontation. Then, after being sequestered in a cubicle to reduce her external stimulation and quiet the ER, Mary quickly proceeded to light a fire in the wastebasket. Even the fire alarms didn't get her attention or drown out her expletives.

When I first entered the room to evaluate Mary, she lifted up her dress and started thrusting her pelvis in wild gyrations, shouting profanities. Mary hadn't slept in a week; she was disheveled, dirty, and totally out of control. She was clearly a danger to herself and others. Although I was only twenty-five years old, I was the psychiatric resident on call and I had to make decisions quickly about her treatment.

It wasn't easy, but we administered intramuscular Thorazine (an antipsychotic medication) and other sedatives, and admitted her to the locked psychiatric unit. Unfortunately, we did need to use soft, safe physical restraints until we could calm her down, but Mary responded well after the emergency pharmaceutical intervention.

Any medical crisis, whether it's a heart attack, a physical trauma, a stroke, acute asthma, or what have you, requires the best emergency medical care we have in our repertoire, whether it is intravenous drugs or an urgent surgical procedure. Psychiatric emergencies such as mania, severe depression, or a suicide attempt are as life-threatening as any other medical emergency. In psychiatric emergencies, the safety of the patient as well as those around them is always paramount.

Mary required significant pharmaceutical intervention to help her bring her unpredictable and explosive behavior under control. When she arrived at the emergency room, the physiology in her brain was such that she was not "in her right mind" and needed protection from her own self. But are there times when stable medical conditions may best be treated alternatively? I believe so.

While pharmaceuticals are important in emergency and mainstream medicine, the overzealous use of drugs is also a problem. For example, did you know that the fourth-leading cause of death in the United States today is adverse reactions to drugs that are properly prescribed by physicians? That's right, *properly*: the right drug for the right reason, and still such a disheartening statistic! Clearly, a better answer for physicians is to understand even more about the cellular biology of the disease and the biochemical processes that cause symptoms. This is where the integrative approach comes in.

Nutraceutical and metabolic support is a new emerging science that allows us physicians to offer safer modalities in the treatment of stable patients. In cardiology, for example, I employ a metabolic approach in which vital nutrients are given to patients to help facilitate enzymatic and metabolic reactions in the direction of healing and recovery. When treatments are aimed at the metabolic and mitochondrial level of biochemical disorders, then patients can truly be helped, and with the guidance of their physicians, many patients can become less reliant on medication—or, in some instances, weaned off drugs completely. They must always be on the alert, however, for any symptoms, such as chest discomfort or pain, which indicate that it is time to be reevaluated, whether they are on medications, natural therapies, or a combination.

Healing Depression & Bipolar Disorder Without Drugs offers physicians and patients a similar plan for psychiatric problems, suggesting more natural approaches to depression and BPD that may be considered when the affected person's condition has been stable for some time. And, just like my cardiac patients, the person with depression or BPD who is using a pharmaceutical, natural, or combined treatment plan, as well as his or her family, can be educated about any symptoms that warrant reevaluation and possible medical intervention.

Even as youngsters, my siblings and I could tell when Dad was becoming manic or starting to show symptoms of an emerging depression. The problem with BPD is that a patient must be in a relationship with someone he trusts to give him feedback, whether it's a family member or a frequently seen therapist. Early mania is a state of feeling "good" for the person with BPD, so he is not likely to seek help unless he has specific guidelines, like noticing that he is sleeping less, spending money, and so on. Still, a person with BPD is not likely to notice the early signs at all. If you have depression or BPD and want to stop taking pharmaceutical drugs, you must work with health professionals who are willing to substitute nutraceutical and other supports while you are under their care.

Health care professionals who are comfortable treating patients from the nutraceutical point of view have learned that these applications can be truly rewarding in relieving the discomfort of their patients. Physicians who choose to use an integrative approach find it offers them and their patients the best of both worlds, allowing them to choose between pharmaceutical and nutraceutical interventions to limit side effects and improve quality of life.

Healing Depression & Bipolar Disorder Without Drugs can be a vital resource for those health professionals who wish to treat mental illness from the integrative point of view. Gracelyn Guyol explores challenging questions about how people become mentally ill. How much do mercury and other heavy metals, parasites, thyroid dysfunction, electrolyte abnormalities, and other entities contribute to symptoms? When might they even be the major contributing factor? How does one even check for these variables? The answers to these newer questions will take us years to find, but the work of identifying them is clearly offered here in a straightforward manner by someone who has been on her own search for answers as part of her own path to healing.

This book raises other intriguing questions. Can metabolic support and the eradication of toxins, insecticides, pesticides, heavy metals, *candida*, microbes, herpes, Epstein-Barr virus, and others help reduce the onset of physical and mental illness? And can treatment with biochemical supports such as vitamins, minerals, essential sugars, amino acids, coenzyme Q_{10}, and essential fatty acids like the omega-3s, to mention a few, enhance quality of life?

Ms. Guyol mentions some really good forms of alternative healing for the reader. I was particularly impressed with the section on essential sugars, a new area of medical interest that may offer more treatment modalities in the future. (I would add that although it is not discussed here, D-ribose is an outstanding natural sugar that's new and effective in the field of cardiology and in the future may be found to be equally important for treating mental health issues.)

Whatever approaches are employed, patients, families, and health practitioners must work as a team. *Healing Depression & Bipolar Disorder Without Drugs* should be read not only by patients but also by the health professionals who treat depression and bipolar disorder on a day-to-day basis. I believe that if someone with a chronic mental illness wishes to try an integrative approach, and if he or she finds a willing health care provider with an open mind, then miracles can occur in the healing process.

The strongest aspect of this book is that it offers hope to patients with bipolar disorder, a biochemical anomaly that is poorly understood. In this country, there is often a terrible stigma for those afflicted with mental illness, and it's one that can be lifted with the kind of educational reading found in this text. This book provides the raw materials for both the patient and the mental health provider to create a more fulfilling and healthy way of living.

—*Stephen T. Sinatra, M.D., F.A.C.C., author of* The Sinatra Solution

Why Drugs Are Not the Best Solution for Mental Disorders

Depression is the leading cause of disability globally. In the United States, it affects roughly 18 million adults, twice as many women as men, and ranks just behind high blood pressure as the most common chronic medical condition.[1] Yet millions more cases are never diagnosed because people are reluctant to seek medical help, fearing the tremendous stigma attached to mental illness, or they do not realize they are ill because symptoms can range from mild lethargy to powerful feelings of hopelessness and despair. About two-thirds of those who commit suicide are depressed at the time of their death.[2]

Bipolar disorder occurs in roughly 2.6 percent of the population, men and women equally.[3] It was once called manic-depression because moods swing between manic highs and depressive lows in widely varying cycles. Highs can range from slightly elevated, carefree moods to dangerous euphoria, mixed with anxiety, anger, and occasional rage, before plunging into depression. Bipolar disorder is especially frightening because conventional medicine has not figured out what causes these random cycles or how to consistently control them. Viewed as having a lifelong "incurable" illness, many bipolar patients are unable to hold jobs, are frequently institutionalized, or live in a psychiatric drug–induced haze. Twenty-five to 50 percent of bipolar patients attempt suicide at least once, and if untreated, have a 15 percent higher risk of death from suicide than the overall population.[4]

Medications used to treat these disorders sometimes cause such horrible side effects that many patients hate their "meds," and many discontinue use. Some patients self-medicate with alcohol, tobacco, caffeine, chocolate, sugar, and street drugs—especially when disorders are undiagnosed. They use any substance that makes them temporarily feel good. Ironically, these choices increase brain dysfunction and contribute to addiction, crime, and obesity. Other patients continue taking prescribed medications, suffering serious, even life-altering side effects, unaware that there are alternatives.

Treatment of my own bipolar disorder stands as a sobering example. Although my lifelong episodes of depression were first diagnosed in the 1980s, the manic side was not noticed until 1993, when symptoms became more pronounced with age. I refused lithium because it had not helped my mother and I had witnessed its numerous adverse side effects. Given another commonly prescribed antidepressant that also helps control mood swings, my life immediately became easier and less stressful. Between 1994 and 1995, however, I began growing breast cysts and tumors so rapidly that I had surgery twice in twelve months. Following each operation, more growths developed.

Anxious to figure out the cause of these growths, I consulted a naturopathic doctor who prescribed an anti-inflammatory diet that slowed the proliferation of cysts. I next focused on systematically ridding myself of all possible toxins, because cellular mutation can be caused in part by foreign molecules, like those in psychiatric medications. By the time another tumor appeared in 1998, the only unnatural substance I was still using was the antidepressant.

The psychiatrist who had prescribed the drug consulted available reports that showed the medication caused mammary tumors in mice, although results were deemed inconclusive since the rodents received nine thousand times the dose given a human (adjusted for relative weight). This "clue" came on the heels of my two years of research and elimination of toxins. Since the growths had appeared roughly a year after I began taking the antidepressant, I decided to taper off the drug to see what would happen. My bipolar symptoms had always been relatively mild, so my life would not be in danger without medication, but it might be from cancer.

Within two months, the latest tumor had disappeared and no new growths had emerged. I had discovered many other unadvertised but well-documented health risks from antidepressants during my combing of popular and professional literature. Refusing *all* psychiatric medications, I resolved to end my bipolar cycles without drugs.

In November 1999, I consulted a brain research center where two genetic conditions were identified that contributed to my mental imbalances (see chapter 1 for details). Within four months of taking only vitamins and minerals prescribed by the center to compensate for these genetic "errors," my manic cycles ended.

However, the depression continued and, no longer relieved by mania, worsened. I researched and tried many promising treatments, but nothing provided permanent relief. Finally in 2001, I read a new book on clinical trials of omega-3 fatty acids, found in inexpensive fish oils, which showed that they were helpful in treating bipolar disorder. Within a couple of days of taking three grams of these good fats daily, my depression lifted.

Tremendously relieved to be free of chaotic mood swings and the fear of breast cancer, I decided to share all I had learned. I began writing, lecturing, and organizing seminars on healing without drugs. After I went public with my story, dozens of strangers sought me out, confiding that they or a loved one also struggled with depression or bipolar illness. Understanding and advice from another who had "been there" seemed to give great comfort, direction, and hope.

In 2004, I spoke on a Recovery Panel at Non-Pharma III, an alternative mental health conference in California organized by Safe Harbor.[5] There I met and interviewed many others who had ended a wide variety of mental disorders without the use of pharmaceuticals. Each story was unique but had one common thread: We did not just *treat* our mental illness, we *cured* it—eliminating the symptoms—a feat no drug could claim.

Diagnosis

Feeling "sad" or "blue" following the death of a loved one, the loss of a job, a traumatic experience, a divorce, or some other overwhelming stress is a normal, healthy reaction that time often heals. Harder to understand is what triggers depression or manic highs when there is no obvious cause.

Long a mystery, how the brain operates has become one of the most rapidly expanding frontiers of medical science today, thanks primarily to technological advances. Positron emission tomography (PET) is the most exciting of these because it allows imaging a *living* brain in action, making processes observable. Magnetic resonance imaging (MRI) offers a view of brain cysts, tumors, and changes in neuron activity in different regions as they are affected by thoughts and emotions, with better spatial resolution than PET. X-ray computerized tomography (CT) scans provide a view of the brain's structure but not its functioning. Most mental patients, unfortunately, do not have access to such expensive testing unless tumors or similar physiological causes are suspected.

Depression and bipolar disorder are syndromes, diagnosed based on a cluster of symptoms, presumably related, that collectively indicate a psychological disorder or disturbance. Thus, a listing of the patient's mental and emotional difficulties is still the cornerstone of all diagnoses. A therapist will typically take a patient's psychiatric and medical history, noting any mental illnesses in the patient's parents, siblings, and children. Symptoms and differences between major depression, mild or episodic depressions, and bipolar disorder in adults and children are set out below:

Major Depression

5 or more symptoms for at least 2 weeks

Onset may be abrupt

Mood is not dependent on external factors

SYMPTOMS

Fatigue, slow speech and actions

Persistently sad, hopeless, pessimistic mood

Poor concentration

Loss of interest or pleasure in life

Low self-esteem, low self-confidence

Indecisive, easily overwhelmed

Significant change in appetite/weight

Insomnia or oversleeping

Reduced libido

Restlessness, irritability, excessive crying

Feeling worthless or inappropriate guilt

Substance abuse

Thoughts of death or suicide

Often unable to function

Mild Depression (also called Dysthymia)

Milder but more chronic form of depression

Onset gradual, often in adolescence

SYMPTOMS

Same as major depression but fewer in number and milder

External events trigger mood changes

Usually able to function and not normally suicidal

May have persistent physical symptoms: digestive upset,
headaches, etc.

Postpartum Depression

"The baby blues" following childbirth

Caused by a drop in progesterone and other hormonal imbalances after giving birth

Symptoms resemble those of major depression

"Secondary" Depression

Symptoms of depression brought on by serious medical problems—cancer, diabetes, heart attack, AIDS, etc.

Seasonal Affective Disorder (SAD)

Depression in the winter when length of day shortens; also triggered by shift work, jet lag, or being confined indoors with little natural light

----

Source: American Psychiatric Association Practical Guidelines for the Treatment of Psychiatric Disorders (Washington, DC: American Psychiatric Association, 2000), 453.

Bipolar Disorder I & II

Periods of major depression interspersed with episodes of mania

Bipolar I is a more severe form, with full manic episodes that may include hallucinations and delusions

Bipolar II patients have more symptoms of depression and identification of mania may even be delayed

Onset is frequently in young adulthood

Moods not usually related to external events

MANIA SYMPTOMS

Extremely silly, optimistic, euphoric, or irritable moods

Volatile anger, aggression, agitation

Inflated self-esteem, confidence, grandeur

Decreased need for sleep

Bizarre, racing thoughts or ideas

Rapid or excessive speech

Lack of focus, distractibility, or hyperfocus

Impulsive, risky behavior

Excessive spending

Promiscuity, hypersexuality

Substance abuse

Highly impaired ability to function

Source: Johns Hopkins Symptoms & Remedies (New York: Medletter Association, 1999), 344;
Current Medical Diagnoses & Treatment (New York: McGraw-Hill, 2004), 1029.

According to the National Mental Health Association, one in thirty-three children and one in eight adolescents may have depression. One in five children have a diagnosable mental, emotional, or behavioral disorder, with attention deficit hyperactivity disorder (ADHD) the most common. Nearly one-fourth of children with ADHD have or will develop bipolar disorder, according to a study reported in the *Journal of the American Academy of Child and Adolescent Psychiatry* in 1996.[6]

How to Differentiate Between Attention Deficit Hyperactivity Disorder (ADHD) and Bipolar Disorder (BD) in Children

ADHD children are destructive from carelessness or inattention; BD children exhibit severe temper tantrums with manic physical and emotional energy and may be openly sadistic.

Outburst duration differs: ADHDs calm down in 20–30 minutes; BD tantrums may last up to four hours.

"Regression" during angry episodes is rarely seen in ADHD but common in BD; also, a BD child may have little memory of the tantrum.

Misbehavior in ADHD is often accidental; in BD it is frequently intentional.

Depression is not a predominant symptom in ADHD children, but prominent with BD.

Irritability is prominent in BD children, especially in the morning, but not in ADHD.

OTHER CHILDHOOD BIPOLAR SYMPTOMS

Gifted abilities, especially verbal and artistic

Insatiable craving for sweets and carbohydrates

Risk seeker

Gross distortions in reality or interpretation of emotional events

Sleep disturbances and/or severe nightmares, often graphically violent with gore

Symptoms may be accompanied by bed-wetting, night terrors, separation anxiety, panic and phobias, and learning disabilities.

Source: C. Popper, M.D., "Diagnosing Bipolar vs. ADHD," *Newsletter of the American Academy of Child and Adolescent Psychiatric* (Summer 1989): 5–6.

In adults, symptoms of major depression often closely mimic those of early Alzheimer's, since depression severely impairs both memory and the ability to think clearly. People with either condition often speak slowly with long pauses or have a vacant stare, and their physical movements are slowed. While depression has uneven progression over a relatively short period of weeks, Alzheimer's shows steady progression over months or years. Even more revealing, depressed people readily complain about their inability to concentrate or their memory loss, whereas Alzheimer's patients tend to deny that anything untoward has occurred.

Other emotional and personality disorders—anxiety, anorexia, bulimia, paranoia, obsessive-compulsive disorders—may appear concurrently with depression or bipolar disorder. For instance, I experienced attention deficit disorder (ADD) and SAD along with my mania and depression; some people have obsessions and compulsions, bulimia, or delusions that overlap with bipolar symptoms. Any mix of mental symptoms may result from the causes covered in chapters 1–8, but each ailment has its own idiosyncrasies. The primary focus of this book will be on depression and bipolar disorder only.

How the Nervous System and Brain Affect Mood Disorders

Our two-part nervous system has a tremendous impact on mental health. The central nervous system, consisting of the brain and spinal cord, regulates body activity by processing and coordinating nerve signals. The peripheral nervous system includes nerves that emerge from the brain and spinal cord, branching throughout the body, controlling voluntary actions (such as walking) and involuntary actions (such as heartbeat).

Neurons are the signaling units of the nervous system. Composed of a cell body, one or two long nerve fibers called axons, and numerous branching dendrites, neurons transmit messages in the form of electrical impulses from one cell to another. A chemical message—or neurotransmitter—is converted into an electrical impulse when it's picked up by a dendrite. It moves through the cell body, then travels down the fiber. This electrical impulse then changes back into a chemical and is propelled across a small gap, called a synapse, in a process that takes less than 1/5,000th of a second, allowing the brain to react instantaneously to stimuli.[7, 8]

Neurotransmitters are produced from specific amino acids found in protein. Although more than one hundred neurotransmitters have been identified so far, only a few are known to figure in depression, mania, and other moods when deficiencies occur. Those basic neurotransmitters, the substances from which they are made, and some of their actions are outlined in the table.

Neurotransmitters for Mental Health

NEUROTRANSMITTER; PRECURSOR NEEDED	ACTION	WHAT ITS DEFICIENCY CAUSES
Serotonin, from tryptophan	The primary "feel good" source; also initiates sleep, controls pain	Depression, anxiety, irritability, insomnia, phobias, substance abuse, eating disorders, cravings for sweets and carbohydrates
Acetylcholine, from choline, oxygen, & glucose	Improves memory, mental alertness; triggers muscle action in nerve cells	Fatigue, depression, poor concentration and recall, loss of brain speed
Dopamine, from tyrosine or phenylalanine	Controls physical movement; improves mood, energy, sex drive, memory, immune function; stimulates growth hormone to burn fat, builds muscle, regulates body temperature	Parkinson's disease, depression, low motivation, inability to complete tasks (too much dopamine contributes to mania)
GABA (gamma-aminobutyric acid) from	"Inhibitory" or calming effect on nervous system; curbs chronic	Anxiety, tension, panic, insomnia, substance abuse (low levels

NEUROTRANSMITTER: PRECURSOR NEEDED (CONT.)	ACTION (CONT.)	WHAT ITS DEFICIENCY CAUSES (CONT.)
glutamic acid or glutamine	stress response; controls release of dopamine in the brain	of GABA may also cause low dopamine symptoms)
Histamine, from histidine	In all nerve cells, impacts mood, appetite, sleep, and thought; speeds up metabolism; essential to immunity; (dopamine and epinephrine modulate histamine release)	Hallucinations, paranoia, grandiosity; (high levels cause allergies, addictions, obsession/compulsion, depression, suicide)
Norepinephrine, (also called noradrenaline) from tyrosine & phenylalanine	A hormone that also acts as a neurotransmitter; is "excitatory," causing alertness, pleasure, motivation, euphoria; vital in carrying short-term memories to long-term storage; stimulates metabolic rate	Depression, low sex drive, disrupted sleep

The Rise of Psychiatric Pharmaceuticals

Drugs are now *the* major tools for treating mental illness. The first tranquilizers, introduced in 1952, have been followed nearly every decade since by a new class of psychiatric drugs. Selective serotonin reuptake inhibitors, or SSRIs, are the latest class. They work by preventing the body from reabsorbing used serotonin, leaving more available in the synapse. SSRIs were introduced with great hope and hype, but their risks or side effects, if mentioned at all, were and still are in tiny print on the package insert and trivialized by manufacturers, even to prescribing physicians.

Psychiatric drugs were a godsend compared to past therapies. Patients unlucky enough to be institutionalized before the 1900s were caged, starved, whipped, or, worse, treated like dangerous beasts. In the 1930s, *standard* asylum medicine included induced insulin coma, electroshock, and lobotomy, primarily because these made patients more compliant, less dangerous to their keepers. Not coincidentally, these treatments were also very lucrative for practitioners.

The cornerstone of modern pharmacology was slowly laid in the second half of the nineteenth century. Built on the work of Claude Bernard, a French founder of experimental medicine, and Paul Ehrlich, a German Nobel Prize winner for his studies of immunity, it was British physiologist John Langley who first formulated the hypothesis that drugs interact with specific receptors on cells. Only after fifty years of ongoing research, however, were psychiatric drugs introduced, and it has taken another fifty years for drugs to become the dominant protocol.

In 2004, the Mayo Clinic's Web site said of bipolar disorder, "Its causes are elusive, and there's no cure." Yet many doctors on the frontiers of research believe otherwise. Distinguished scientists often disagree because revolutionary changes are generally slow to be widely implemented. For instance, disc brakes were invented in 1901 but did not become standard equipment until the 1980s—and liquid crystal displays now seen on watches, televisions, and cell phones were first discovered in 1888.[9]

Why did it take so long for drugs to become the treatment of choice for psychiatric conditions? Perhaps because of the limited scientific evidence of pharmaceuticals' true advantage over psychotherapy or placebos. A placebo is an inactive substance given to participants in clinical tests so all study participants believe that they are taking the drug, thus creating a "control" group. When applying to the Food and Drug Administration (FDA) for approval, manufacturers of new drugs only have to provide *two* studies that demonstrate a "statistically significant" improvement in patients taking the drug compared to the control group. In 1999, an agency in the Department of Health and Human Services did an analysis of data from more than eighty clinical studies of the newer antidepressants. They found that half the patients did not respond to the drugs at all. Of the half who did respond, 64 percent of the benefit was attributed to the placebo effect, a benefit that arises from the patient's expectation of healing rather than from the actual treatment.[10]

Earlier short-term studies, in the 1980s and 1990s, had found that two-thirds of patients responded equally well to psychotherapy and medication. But long-term studies that tracked patients up to four years gave the advantage to psychotherapy, showing that patients on drugs alone relapsed more readily. However, drugs were faster, easier, and less expensive (or so it seemed at the time), so insurers began to limit payments for psychotherapy visits and doctors began to recommend that patients stay on drugs indefinitely.[11]

Within two decades, the pharmaceutical industry became astoundingly profitable, thanks in no small part to government programs like Medicare and Medicaid paying for antidepressants and other psychiatric drugs. By 2001, the ten U.S. drug companies on the Fortune 500 list had profits of 18.5 percent of sales, compared to average profits of 3.3 percent of sales for companies in the other Fortune 500 industries combined. According to Marcia Angell, M.D., in *The Truth About the Drug Companies*, such stupendous wealth enabled the industry to "co-opt every institution" that might protect the consumer, "including the U.S. Congress, the Food and Drug Administration, academic medical centers, and the medical profession itself."[12]

Such extraordinary profits created an environment that allows abuses in clinical trials and condones blatant conflicts of interest among FDA staff and doctors serving on investigative panels. It enables the drug industry to buy off researchers who plan to publish studies showing negative results (such as suicidal tendencies) of some antidepressants, to "educate" doctors by paying for lavish trips and entertainment; and to hire hundreds of academic experts to publish research articles glorifying antidepressants and advocating their long-term use.[13]

Awash in drug advertising revenues, the media cannot be expected to bite this affluent hand and warn consumers about the dangers of these drugs. No organization or group has even 1 percent of the pharmaceutical industry's budget to counter misinformation or give consumers and doctors a more balanced perspective. Thus, the primary treatment offered to depressed or bipolar people today is drugs—period.

Dangers of Psychiatric Drugs

Because every patient's biochemistry is unique, each person reacts to a drug differently, so doctors prescribe most on a trial-and-error basis, attempting to find one that relieves symptoms with minimal side effects. Yet, drugs do not work for 50 percent of mental patients,[14] and more than 50 percent of those for whom they *do* work discontinue use due to side effects.[15]

When single drugs fail, untested "cocktails" are tried, using lithium, SSRIs, sedatives, or tranquilizers in an endless variety of combinations. If these also fail to provide relief, patients despair and become deeply disillusioned, feeling "used" by an industry that seems to care more about profits than making people well. Some doctors are just as disillusioned as their patients, but, untrained in any other method, they continue offering the newest drug, desperately hoping it will induce mental stability.

Both consumers and doctors are under the impression that medications are thoroughly tested prior to FDA approval, but most clinical trials last for only six to eight *weeks*—too short a period for many side effects to emerge—and are anything but scientific, according to some researchers. More than 50 percent of drugs approved by the

FDA between 1976 and 1985 were found, during or after marketing, to have previously undetected "serious" negative side effects, according to the Government Accounting Office in 1990.[16] Critics say the industry's clinical trials meet the minimal FDA requirements, but do not stand up to the rigors of genuine science.[17]

Clinical trials of psychiatric drugs include hundreds of people recruited from around the country, but trials deliberately exclude anyone with severe or complicated emotional problems and those who are physically ill, actively suicidal, or taking other drugs. In other words, the trials leave out a population very much like those who will be using the drugs.[18] Plus, drugs are almost never tested on patients in combination with other psychiatric medications, although they are very commonly prescribed that way.

The latest class, the SSRIs, were marketed as a breakthrough because they are "selective" for serotonin, a description creating the impression that because of this selectivity they were somehow safer than older drugs.[19] That impression does not match reality, according to Joseph Glenmullen, M.D., in *Prozac Backlash*.

SSRI antidepressants block "reuptake" of serotonin, that is, removal of the neurotransmitter from the space between nerve cells. Artificially elevated levels of serotonin cause the system to become hyperactive. The brain attempts to compensate by *reducing* the cells' sensitivity to serotonin, a process known as "downregulation," and makes other long-term adaptations to overcome the drug's effects that may permanently alter DNA with totally unknown consequences.[20]

Neurotransmitters like serotonin do not operate independently—they are linked through complex circuitry to other neurotransmitters, such as epinephrine and dopamine. According to Dr. Glenmullen, after a decade of SSRI use, doctors and researchers are just beginning to understand how these systems interact. Boosting serotonin levels, it turns out, triggers a drop in dopamine. Low levels of dopamine contribute to Parkinson's disease as well as other serious side effects.[21]

Tics (sometimes permanent, disfiguring muscle spasms) were first associated with the use of an earlier class of drugs, tranquilizers, and are believed to be the result of slow, progressive brain damage that manifests itself only when it becomes severe.[22] Side effects of SSRI antidepressants are similar to but milder than those of tranquilizers. Glenmullen says the "critical variable determining the degree of [brain] damage appears to be *total cumulative exposure* to the drugs."[23] Some scientists are concerned that silent brain damage from SSRIs may be occurring but will not become obvious for another decade, when it is epidemic and too late.

Almost as frightening, pharmaceutical companies are expanding market share by promoting antidepressants for children, totally disregarding what is known, and the massive amount that is unknown, about how neurotransmitters and growth hormones interact. Stimulants (Ritalin, Dexedrine, and others) given to children for attention deficit disorder (ADD) have been proven to stunt children's growth—both their height and weight—because the drugs interfere with the pituitary gland's natural production of human growth hormone.[24] Additionally, a 2002 study showed decreased growth during treatment with SSRIs as well.[25] For this reason, many doctors believe that neither antidepressants nor stimulants should ever be administered to children.

Pregnant women and nursing mothers should be aware that all psychiatric drugs have to be able to cross the blood-brain barrier in order to enter the brain. This capacity enables them to cross the placenta as well and circulate in the fetal bloodstream, entering the fetus's developing brain.[26] The drugs also enter a nursing mother's milk, impacting the infant's brain too.

In spite of this, consumers of all ages have been encouraged to use antidepressants for years, some for relatively minor complaints. One survey showed primary-care doctors rather than psychiatrists write more than 70 percent of prescriptions for Prozac, Zoloft, Paxil, and Luvox, leading one to assume that these drugs are *most often* recommended by doctors who are least aware of their dangers.[27] In order to make appropriate risk/benefit decisions, however, patients, or their families, should be fully informed about these drugs.

Common Side Effects

Patients often receive little advance warning about possible drug side effects or, if they are given literature, they may not read it, believing the percentage of people adversely affected is so tiny that they are not at risk. The drug's benefits, however, are widely advertised and, until recent legal changes, included scant mention of dangers. To many patients, side effects often come as a complete surprise.

Another surprise may be that a drug prescribed to treat initial symptoms of depression or mania may cause new symptoms for which additional psychiatric medications need to be prescribed. It is not unusual for people to be taking two to four psychiatric drugs at once. For this reason, a brief summary of the various classes of these drugs and their potential side effects is included below. Reactions vary by brand and type of drug, of course, and this is a sampling meant to convey the extent of the risks, not a comprehensive list. Hopefully, it will encourage you to look up a specific medication in drug reference books at a local library *before* filling the prescription.

Mild symptoms from SSRI antidepressants include dry mouth, drowsiness or insomnia, dizziness, diarrhea or constipation, headache, and weight gain or loss. According to independent studies, 54–65 percent of patients experience sexual dysfunction, although manufacturers report only 2–5 percent.[28, 29] Less frequent but more severe side effects include increased depression and suicidal tendencies; neurologically driven agitation, ranging from mild leg tapping to severe panic; tics or muscle spasms; and Parkinsonism.[30] Prozac and Luvox increase the risk of inducing mania in children.[31]

Tricyclic antidepressants and atypical antidepressants share many of the SSRI side effects but have others as well. Some atypical antidepressants produce the same problems as tranquilizers, making it doubly important to research your particular drug.[32]

Monoamine oxidase inhibitors (MAOIs) are antidepressants. Less frequently prescribed, they interact with numerous drugs and require patients to avoid foods containing tyramine (red wines, aged cheeses, smoked meats) or risk violent headaches and possible strokes. MAOIs may induce mania, agitation, muscle spasms, elevated body temperature, or delirium.[33]

Lithium, the first drug of choice for bipolar disorder, is notorious for causing weight gain, tremors, drowsiness, dry mouth, nausea, confusion, and restlessness. Less common are blackouts, seizures, loss of coordination, tinnitus (ringing in the ears), blurred vision, vomiting, anorexia, water retention, as well as hypothyroidism, cardiac arrhythmias, skin acne and rashes, hair loss, and birth defects in offspring.[34] After taking lithium for years, many people experience memory problems and find it difficult to work.[35] The *American Psychiatric Association Practice Guidelines* report, "Up to 75 percent of patients treated with lithium experience some side effects."[36]

Mood stabilizers used in place of lithium to control mania or reduce mood swings work primarily through sedation. Those first developed as anticonvulsants can cause tremor, difficulty walking, confusion, delirium, weight gain, stomach upset, and blood-clotting problems. Others may bring on insomnia, anxiety, and addiction as well as compromising liver function.[37]

In the 1980s, tranquilizers were first found to cause tics (disfiguring muscle spasms) in 40 percent of patients—half of which were permanent—and in some cases these tics appeared after only two years of use. Malpractice suits were filed and huge settlements were awarded to patients who had not been warned of the dangers. Tranquilizers were then separated into two categories, calling the more dangerous ones "major" tranquilizers, while sedatives, like Valium, were dubbed "minor" tranquilizers. Today, major tranquilizers are also called antipsychotics or neuroleptics in what might be viewed as a marketing ploy to disconnect them from these dreaded, often permanent ailments in the minds of prospective patients.[38]

Major tranquilizers cause Parkinsonism, agitation, obesity, and diabetes mellitus.[39] The drugs are required to carry a warning about the

dangers of tardive dyskinesia (irreversible abnormal muscle movements, commonly of face, eyes, mouth, and tongue), estimated to occur at rates of 5–7 percent.[40] They may also cause tardive dystonia
(painful, disfiguring muscle spasms, often of face and neck), and tardive akathisia (irritability and anxiety that compel a person into constant motion).[41] Neuroleptic malignant syndrome can be a fatal side
effect of tranquilizers. Similar to viral brain inflammation, this reaction brings on severe abnormal movements, fever, sweating, and un-
stable blood pressure that can progress to delirium and coma.
Although considered rare, neuroleptic malignant syndrome is estimated to occur in .7–2.5 percent of patients treated with tranquilizers. The FDA considers anything with a rate of 1 percent to be
common.[42]

Minor tranquilizers that are prescribed for anxiety or insomnia
may induce drowsiness, fatigue, confusion, headache, nausea, dizziness, and lack of coordination that may result in falls. Slurred speech,
poor judgment, hallucinations, and behavioral abnormalities are also
common, especially in children or the elderly. Many of these antianx-
iety drugs are highly addictive and subject to abuse.[43]

Facts About and Dangers of Psychiatric Drugs

50% of depressed and bipolar patients are not helped by
    antidepressants[44]

50% stop taking psychiatric medications due to side effects[45]

21% using lithium relapse within two years[46]

85% of those who recover from a major depressive disorder
    experience a recurrence[47]

58% experience sexual dysfunction from antidepressants[48]

40% develop tics from use of tranquilizers (50% of which are
    permanent)[49]

1% of adults using Prozac become manic[50]

6% of children on Prozac dropped out of a study due to mania; 4% of children on Luvox had manic reactions[51]

Depression and suicidality can worsen from antidepressants, according to a 2004 FDA warning[52]

SSRI antidepressants decrease growth in children[53]

Pharmaceutical industry–funded research that shows drugs are dangerous or ineffective often does not get published, and funding for follow-up studies usually becomes unavailable once a negative finding emerges. Therefore, small studies that do get published, indicating increased health risks, should make consumers extremely wary. The research cited below is not conclusive because study results have not yet been replicated by independent groups of researchers. However, these strongly suggest the possibility of additional unadvertised dangers.

Potential Health Risks from Psychiatric Drugs

Doubled risk of non-Hodgkin's lymphoma from taking as few as 5 prescriptions of tricyclic antidepressants[54]

"Significant" increased risk of invasive ovarian cancer after 6 months use of psychotropic drugs (antidepressants, antipsychotics, sedatives, anticonvulsants, amphetamines)[55]

Poor metabolizers (described in chapter 1) show elevated risk of lung and bladder cancers; Prozac and Paxil inhibit a metabolism gene[56]

Risk of heart attack doubles with tricyclic antidepressant use[57]

Elevated risk for developing Type II diabetes from major tranquilizers[58]

SSRI use associated with development of movement disorders, including Parkinsonism[59]

Slow, long-term brain damage: suspected but as yet unproven

In spite of these dangers, no patient should abruptly stop taking psychiatric medications. Once the brain has adapted to a supply of drugs, whether illegal or prescription, quickly ending the influx may cause unpredictable, life-threatening reactions. Chapter 14 covers the steps to take *before* slowly tapering off drugs under a doctor's care and specifies common withdrawal symptoms that may occur.

A New Approach to Healing

Quietly, with little fanfare, new and better solutions have evolved of which many people are unaware, primarily because inexpensive natural remedies generate slim profits, so they command no massive advertising budgets to promote them to doctors or consumers.

Healing Depression & Bipolar Disorder Without Drugs is written to present viable alternative treatments for depression and bipolar disorder through the stories of individuals who have successfully ended their symptoms. Since most health books are written by doctors, few have tapped the wisdom of patients—those, like me, who have lived with and successfully eradicated a disorder through personal research, trial, and error. I believe these healing anecdotes, when told collectively, offer valuable perspective and insight, a road map for others.

Medical researchers have studied the causes and treatments for bipolar disorder and depression for decades. But professionals tend to do narrow, focused research, seeking solutions aimed at developing salable products. Or they do research to discover a new process or data that will lead to grants, enabling still more research. There is nothing wrong with this. It has provided a foundation of scientific understanding for medicine.

Patients are not bound by the restrictions of researchers, however. We can pursue anything that seems likely to work, test it personally, observing and applying the results. Our only motivation is getting well, usually as inexpensively as possible, and if others follow this approach, we could dramatically reduce out-of-control health care costs.

When a patient's research is successful, however, we simply get on with our lives and nobody knows or benefits from what we have learned.

Healing Depression & Bipolar Disorder Without Drugs is meant to share with readers the patients' perspective and collective, hard-earned knowledge in order to save others time and money in their own quest.

Part I covers the elimination of things that may trigger mental or mood symptoms: medicines, diseases, environmental toxins, flawed digestion, food sensitivities, thyroid or other hormone imbalances, and self-administered agents like alcohol, caffeine, tobacco, and junk food. It tells how to compensate for genetic predispositions with vitamins, minerals, good fats, glyconutrients, enzymes, and amino acids.

Part II identifies natural therapies that have been most successful in rebalancing the brain, releasing traumatic experiences, or increasing the level of neurotransmitters and mind/body communication.

Each chapter opens with the true story of one individual who has ended the symptoms of his or her mental illness without drugs. Those identified by their full names have chosen to become public advocates for change of the current treatment approach to mental health. Others, who prefer privacy, are identified by first name only, a pseudonym.

All are real people. Many have been through a living hell, and I am grateful for their honesty and willingness to share their experience in order to help others. Such accounts show that healing by addressing root causes and repairing the body with natural therapies is not just a nice theory—it is very effective compared to conventional treatments, although not as quick or easy as taking a pill.

The personal accounts are followed by a simple explanation of how underlying causes, nutrients, or therapies impact the brain and body. Understanding *why* and *how* something works in the body helps you choose among the many natural therapy options. It also motivates you to continue the healing regimen even after symptoms are gone.

Part III and the appendices specify how and where to find doctors to assist you and how to begin the healing process covered in parts I and II. Providing the brain with the raw materials it needs for optimum function and eliminating performance-blocking substances brings on heightened mental clarity and energy, usually within a month. Continued over several months, the process can gradually reduce or eliminate depressive or bipolar symptoms. Discovering all the factors contributing to a disorder, however, often takes at least a year or more. Since I had no one to guide me, it took me two years. My hope is that this book will make it an easier, faster, and less uncertain journey for others. The ultimate goal, of course, is to end perpetual drug treatment and *restore mental health*, freeing former patients to create a joyful, fulfilling life.

The natural process discussed in this book will be enhanced by counseling, even after depression and mania symptoms are history. Bipolar cycles foster self-doubt and indecision because one's perspective is always in flux. Depressive patients frequently develop a habitually negative outlook, of which most are unaware. Postrecovery psychotherapy or counseling can help rebuild confidence, break old patterns, and repair the damaged personal relationships that so often lie in the wake of mental illnesses.

Creating optimum brain functioning naturally, instead of relying on dangerous drugs, is a revolution long overdue, but consumers will have to be the driving force behind it. Since 1995, Americans have made more visits to alternative practitioners than to conventional doctors, seeking new healing options, usually for chronic mental and physical conditions that are not alleviated by conventional methods. Only when this startling fact became known did the medical industry suddenly begin talking about "complementary" medicine and changing the medical school curriculum. Given the soaring consumer demand, conventional and alternative medicine will inevitably merge into a more effective system at some time in the future, but if history is any indication, it may take twenty to fifty years. Until this melding occurs, your best option is self-directed health care. Unless patients insist on it, psychiatrists and conventional doctors will never recommend alternative therapies because most have been trained to treat the *symptoms* of illness through drugs or surgery, not to look for and root out underlying *causes*.

Be a catalyst for change. Ask your physician to work *with you* to find a nondrug cure for your depression or bipolar disorder. Pester your insurance company to cover the cost of natural supplements and therapies. Watch your state legislature to make sure these inexpensive natural substances are not outlawed through measures promoted by pharmaceutical companies, most often disguised as safety legislation. Urge congressional representatives to expand government funding for alternative mental health research.

At a time when patients are treated by dozens of specialists with no one in charge of the whole person, you must become that person in charge, a "general contractor" responsible for rebuilding your mental health. When you are well, assist others. Remove the stigma still surrounding mental illness by being open about your condition and your cure, letting others know that they too can find healing without drugs.

PART I

Clearing Potential Underlying Biological Causes

Identifying and Compensating for Genetic Traits

Inexplicable fatigue and depression in my early twenties were diagnosed as hypoglycemia (emotional changes caused by low blood sugar) and I was told to eat plenty of protein snacks. Although I happily grazed, episodes of deep depression plagued me for the next twenty-five years. Many times I attributed them to natural stresses—from going through a divorce, to being a single mother, to founding and running a public relations agency while attempting to build a new house and a relationship with my second husband. Finally in 1993, when I was forty-six years old, a therapist pointed out that the energy highs I experienced between bouts of depression were unusual.

Diagnosed as manic-depressive, or bipolar, I refused lithium, the drug of choice for this illness. It had not worked well for my mother, who had been bipolar all her life but was never diagnosed until she was in her seventies. Lithium made her look puffy, like the Pillsbury Doughboy, and she complained of "cotton mouth," lost her quick chuckle in a flattening of emotions, and developed Parkinson's disease, which ultimately killed her. Instead, I chose Wellbutrin, an antidepressant that helps control mild mood swings. Immediately, my life became easier, less chaotic and stressful.

In 1994, my gynecologist discovered multiple cysts and tumors in my right breast. Since breast cancer is the most common cause of death in women aged forty-five to fifty, I knew others were experiencing this trauma every day, yet nothing prepares you for how it shakes the very foundation of your life. Only after tests revealed that everything was benign did I stop holding my breath about the future. I had surgery twice between 1994 and 1995 to remove growths, but as soon as they were excised, more appeared, like mushrooms after a rain.

My body hadn't done this before. What could be the cause? I had a corps of conventional doctors, but they offered no answer. My gynecologist said he could do nothing except "monitor" the growths until one became malignant and suggested that I see a naturopathic doctor, that dietary changes sometimes helped. Passively waiting for cancer to appear was unthinkable, so I began to research all options.

Friends told me about an exceptional naturopathic doctor (N.D.) named Deirdre O'Connor in the neighboring town of Mystic, Connecticut. Educated in the same basic sciences as medical doctors, naturopaths do postgraduate studies on natural therapies used to prevent or reverse disease and to restore the body's ability to heal. Instead of treating the *symptoms* of disease with drugs or surgery, naturopaths look for ways to eliminate *root causes* of illness, rebuilding and supporting the body's innate healing systems.

Dr. O'Connor told me certain foods stimulate the production of excessive arachidonic acid, which promotes inflammation. This can cause arthritis, stimulate tumor growth, and contribute to cardiac and other degenerative diseases. She suggested that I eliminate the following foods from my diet: dairy products, red meats, refined sugars and flours, margarine, hydrogenated oils, processed foods, alcohol, and wheat and peanuts.

What is left to eat, I asked? She handed me several sheets of instructions (see Anti-Inflammatory Diet, appendix A). I ate fish and organic poultry; three fruits daily, of different colors; four to five vegetables daily, half of them eaten raw for beneficial enzymes; beans and legumes; nuts, seeds, and whole grains (except wheat); "good" omega-3 and -9 fats, found in fish, flaxseed, and olive and nut oils; and drank only herbal teas or filtered water. Dr. O'Connor also prescribed high-potency vitamin and mineral supplements, 1,000 mg of calcium with 500 mg magnesium, 1,000 mg of borage oil, and 1,000 mg of omega-3 fish oils daily.

Terrified of cancer and willing to try anything, I overhauled my eating habits immediately, going straight from her office to the health food store. Within two weeks my energy leveled doubled. I felt fabulous. Three years of severe arthritic pain in both shoulders and up my spine magically disappeared within six weeks. Over the next six months, I lost twenty pounds simply by eating healthy foods. Eliminating all processed foods and cooking only fresh, raw materials was not easy, but motivated by the way I now felt and looked, I persevered.

Next, I systematically eliminated all suspected toxins from my life. Products containing synthetic chemicals—soaps, shampoos, lotions, cosmetics, household cleaning agents—were replaced by natural, plant-derived versions. In summers, I grew food organically without chemical fertilizers or pesticides; in winters, I bought organic foods whenever possible. I drank only tested or filtered water.

Cyst growth slowed, but after eighteen months, another breast tumor appeared. Clearly, diet wasn't the whole answer. Desperate, I read dozens of natural health books, searching for clues in what I came to regard as my giant medical puzzle.

Suddenly, I realized that the growths had appeared a year after I started taking the antidepressant. Could there be a connection? My psychiatrist checked the drug's clinical trials and reported that Wellbutrin appeared to cause mammary tumors in mice, but since the mice were given nine thousand times the amount a human would take relative to body weight, the results were deemed inconclusive. At the breast clinic where I had a biopsy of my new tumor, doctors told me they casually observed that women on antidepressants had more breast discharge than normal, so it was clear that these drugs affected mammary tissue.

While manic-depressive cycles had made my life stressful, I felt lucky. From an outsider's point of view, I functioned "normally." I enjoyed a successful, although stressful, career and had never been institutionalized. Going without the antidepressant would not be life threatening for me, but breast cancer might be.

I tapered off the drug in January 1999. In just two months my tumor disappeared and no new growths emerged. Getting a tumor to go away was a huge victory. I celebrated heartily—until it occurred to me that I faced an even bigger challenge: How would I treat my dysfunctional brain without synthetic chemicals? No doctors I consulted, including my naturopath, knew how to treat bipolar disorder without drugs.

Manic-depressive people have a few advantages, however. We tend to be highly creative—25 percent above normal—and are fearless when manic, believing anything is possible. This aided my career, allowing me to try and often succeed at things more rational people would not have attempted. Over time, I had developed the now-ingrained habit of not limiting myself to what others believed possible. Thus, not finding a doctor who knew how to treat bipolar disorder without pharmaceuticals did not stop me from believing that a non-drug regimen still might be possible.

I had just experienced dramatic proof with my tumor that when the underlying causes of an illness are eliminated, a cure is possible. No drug offered me this hope for my brain. I gave myself two years to find a natural solution.

If the specific brain problems were identified, I felt sure they could be fixed, but who could help me? I read about two researchers—the late Carl Pfeiffer, M.D., and William Walsh, Ph.D.—who had pioneered the use of specific vitamins and minerals to treat all brain chemistry disorders, including depression, bipolar illness, autism, schizophrenia, violence, and attention deficit disorders. In the fall of 1999, I flew to Pfeiffer Treatment Center near Chicago for a consultation.

Pfeiffer Center's assessment of brain chemistry uses analysis of blood, urine, and hair in conjunction with a two-hour medical history. These tests revealed that I had very low zinc and vitamin B_6 levels, stripped from my body by pyroluria, a genetic condition that one 1965 study found in roughly 40 percent of people with mental disorders but only 11 percent of the overall population.[1] Zinc and B_6 are cofactors essential for proper digestion and hundreds of enzymatic processes that ultimately nourish the brain. Low zinc and B_6 also cause elevated histamine and copper levels, which contribute to mania, obsession, or violence. Precise amounts of vitamins and minerals were recommended by the clinic to compensate for this disorder.

Genetic metabolism errors made sense. My Scots/Irish mother had been bipolar all her life; my sister had mild depression; one brother had struggled with alcoholism and occasional rage; another was always overweight in spite of being a vegetarian. I was impressed that Pfeiffer could identify and treat some genetic disorders so readily.

My mania ended after following Pfeiffer's recommendations for four months. Lifting my depression was not so simple, however. Approaching menopause, my hormones were in an uproar. I took Pfeiffer's supplements for fifteen months without relief. I tried herbal therapies, exercise, light therapy, and energy balancing to relieve my depression. Saint-John's-wort did not help. Exercise was the quickest, immediate pick-me-up, and strong sunlight always helped temporarily. An energy healer was able to balance my energies after a few months, but the balance wouldn't hold. Nothing provided a permanent solution—the depression always returned.

Without manic highs, the depression was unrelenting, almost paralyzing. I holed up in my office, working but not productive. There was no joy or laughter in my life. I wanted a divorce, since my husband was always "impossible" from my depressed perspective. Simple tasks, like changing a lightbulb, took three weeks. I avoided friends who required too much energy. As the months dragged on, suicide entered my thoughts for the first time.

At my lowest point, a stranger in Kentucky called to check Pfeiffer's references for a family member stuck in mania. I told him the clinic had quickly ended my mania but confessed that I still struggled with depression. He mentioned two valuable resources: *The Omega-3 Connection*, by Harvard's Andrew Stoll, M.D., and an unrelated Web site, www.truehope.com. Truehope was founded by a man whose wife had committed suicide as a result of bipolar disorder, in spite of the best conventional medicine had to offer. Searching for a natural cure for his bipolar children, he developed a vitamin and mineral supplement that has helped thousands of bipolar patients.

I ordered the book, which described successful clinical trials with thirty bipolar patients using natural fish oils. Since fish oil supplements were already part of my diet, I had some in the refrigerator. Participants in the clinical trials took ten grams daily of EPA (eicosapentaenoic acid), the element in fish oil that affects mood, but Dr. Stoll's book said five grams might be sufficient. I decided to start with three grams a day and see what happened.

Within forty-eight hours, my depression lifted. It was as if a switch had been flipped. Thrilled but cautious, uncertain that it would last, I waited a few months and then began enthusiastically telling everyone about this amazing *natural* antidepressant that ended both my deep depression and seasonal affective disorder (SAD).

With ordinary fish oils, I took eighteen capsules a day to get three grams of EPA. Using Dr. Stoll's Omega Brite brand (filtered of toxins, with seven times more EPA than other brands), I took only six capsules daily, costing $60 a month (which the unenlightened insurance industry did not cover, of course, preferring to pay twice that amount for antidepressants). After a couple of years, when my body's levels of these essential oils were replenished, I switched to a less expensive brand of capsules (still filtered) and recently found a liquid form flavored with orange essential oil made by Pharmax,[2] costing $30 a month. I have been free of all depression, even in winters, since 2002.

Today, I continue to focus on healing the underlying digestive disorders that contributed to my mood swings, lowered my immunity, and will accelerate the aging process. I remain on the anti-inflammatory diet described in appendix A. Supplements taken daily include a high-potency vitamin and mineral supplement; extra B_6 and zinc to offset my pyroluria; capsules of betaine hydrochloride and pepsin with meals (to increase stomach acid) for improved digestion and absorption of nutrients; 3,000 mg of vitamin C; alpha-lipoic acid and other antioxidant supplements for cellular protection and energy; glyconutrients (see chapter 4) to improve cellular communication and boost my immune system; and 1,000–3,000 mg of filtered fish oil. I eat a small amount of protein at every meal. I never skip breakfast, eating healthy snacks whenever I'm hungry but not more than once every two hours, to avoid elevating insulin levels that create the sensation of hunger. I meditate fifteen minutes in the morning, which clears my head and keeps me focused throughout the day. For physical activity, I walk thirty to forty minutes five days a week or swim, play tennis, dance, or garden in season—things I consider fun, not work.

Inborn Genetic Errors

The genetic component of mental illness has long been suspected, based on how frequently mood disorders strike in successive generations of certain families. First-degree relatives—parents, siblings, and children—of a person with bipolar disorder, for instance, are approximately seven times more likely to develop the illness than the rest of the population.[3] By the late 1990s, the long search for a single defective gene had given way to an understanding that multiple gene variants, interacting with unknown environmental risk factors, accounted for many psychiatric disorders.

According to Dr. Elias Zerhouni, director of the National Institutes of Health (NIH), "In 2001, Medicaid paid for more than 50 percent of the total spending on atypical antipsychotics, amounting to $2.7 billion," a figure that had grown 25 percent a year for the previous three years. As a result, NIH has made research on genetic causes of schizophrenia, depression, anxiety, and bipolar disorder a priority.[4]

The National Institute of Mental Health (NIMH) Human Genetics Initiative has compiled the world's largest registry of families affected by schizophrenia, bipolar disorder, and Alzheimer's disease. Currently, scientists from the fields of molecular and cellular biology, genetics, epidemiology, and cognitive and behavioral science have been working together to gain a comprehensive view of factors that influence mood and behavior. It is a huge undertaking to disentangle all the variables and figure out what they mean in terms of brain functioning and mood.

By 2003 NIH-underwritten studies had discovered twelve genes associated with schizophrenia; this discovery was named "breakthrough of the year" by the prestigious journal *Science*. That same year, research at the University of California San Diego School of Medicine identified a specific gene that causes bipolar disorder in certain patients. A mutation in that gene is believed to cause the disorder in perhaps 10 percent of cases. Researchers hypothesize that the mutation creates a hypersensitivity to the neurotransmitter dopamine, leading to mood extremes.[5]

In one 2005 study, blood RNA (ribonucleic acid) from patients diagnosed with schizophrenia or bipolar disorder and control subjects was analyzed. Each disease showed a "unique expressed genome signature," allowing researchers to discriminate between the groups.[6] Blood cell–derived RNA may someday aid in diagnosis of these illnesses.

Most of these studies are impenetrable to anyone except other researchers, but much is being learned. Perhaps within a decade or two, genetic therapy for healing mental disorders will become possible. With the complex interactions of thirty thousand genes and their 3 billion units of DNA (deoxyribonucleic acid, the carrier of genetic information), however, gene therapy may prove to be an impossible dream.[7]

Those suffering now need not passively wait for a scientific breakthrough. In *The Second Brain*, Michael Gershon, M.D., describes how, in animal research, certain genes are "knocked out" when selecting a characteristic one wants an animal to inherit. Much to scientists' surprise, the elimination of many genes thought to be absolutely essential for life had no discernible consequences. The ability of genes to compensate was ". . . prodigious. Take out one gene and others may find a different way to accomplish what the knocked-out gene used to do."

In *Feed Your Genes Right*, author Jack Challem, a nutritional reporter, says "[G]ene activity depends on a variety of nutrients as co-factors. Nutrients provide the building blocks of genes, and they turn many genes on and off."[8] The patient accounts of healing in subsequent chapters often mention family members who also suffer from a mood disorder, indicating a genetic factor. Although only two of the individuals cited here had their genetic condition diagnosed, all nevertheless found healing by simply taking high levels of vitamins, minerals, amino acids, or other substances that provided plenty of raw materials that allowed the body to compensate for genetic errors.

Thus, you don't need to identify genetic flaws in order for your body to work around them. All the cells need are optimum levels of certain raw materials.

Pfeiffer Treatment Center

A few genetic errors associated with mental illness have been identified over the past fifty years and treated with natural supplements by pioneers such as the late Carl Pfeiffer, M.D., a specialist in schizophrenia, and William J. Walsh, Ph.D., a brain chemistry researcher in violent behavior and director of Pfeiffer Treatment Center.

Walsh obtained his Ph.D. in chemical engineering, was a researcher and section head at Argonne National Laboratory for twenty years, holds six patents, and has published more than 175 articles on brain chemistry. After a decade of collaboration with the late Dr. Pfeiffer, Dr. Walsh founded a clinic near Chicago in 1989, naming it Pfeiffer Treatment Center (PTC) in his friend's honor, and an affiliated research wing, Health Research Institute, to enable collaboration between biochemists and medical doctors.[9]

Since his early focus was on violence, Walsh did volunteer work in Illinois prisons in the 1970s, where he found that many inmates had competent, loving families, every educational opportunity, and siblings who were model citizens. He wondered if biological errors might contribute to sociopathic behavior and if the body chemistries of inmates were different from those of average people.

This led to a revealing study of twenty-four pairs of brothers (replicated in three blind, controlled experiments), one average and one violent. The study showed two distinctive patterns in the brain chemistry of violent individuals that were not found in their sibling. Type 1 had an elevated copper/zinc ratio; depressed levels of sodium, potassium, and manganese; and abnormal levels of calcium, magnesium, and blood histamines. Type 2 showed very depressed levels of copper; highly elevated levels of sodium and potassium; elevated levels of blood histamines, kryptopyrroles, lead, cadmium, iron, calcium, and magnesium; and depressed levels of zinc and manganese.

Those with Type 1 levels exhibited Jekyll-Hyde behavior, including episodic violence, poor stress control, and genuine remorse. They often had acne and allergies, and were academic underachievers. Type 2s were assaultive without remorse, they were pathological liars who had a fascination with fire, they were cruel to people and animals, and they often had sleep disorders. Researchers later identified two additional subgroups: nonassaultive delinquents who were impulsive, irritable, underweight underachievers in school and nonassaultive delinquents with sugar cravings, drowsiness, and depression.

Pfeiffer Treatment Center has treated thousands of people with bipolar disorder, depression, schizophrenia, autism, attention deficit, and other disorders, along with behavioral, emotional, and learning problems. Its database includes the brain chemistry profiles of over seventeen thousand patients with mental health problems, including many serial killers.

Pfeiffer Treatment Center tests for four common genetic errors that contribute to mental illness: pyrrole disorder, overmethylation, undermethylation, and metal metabolism. Although the center does not test for it, celiac disease is emerging as another common, undiagnosed genetic ailment. All lead to malfunctions of body systems that support the brain and impact mood.

Pyroluria

In 1958, urine from psychiatric patients was observed to have a mauve tint. A Canadian scientist was the first to identify that the tint was caused by kryptopyrrole molecules. This mauve factor became associated with psychosis when it was found in twenty-seven of thirty-nine schizophrenic patients in 1961. A 1965 study showed the kryptopyrrole molecules in only 11 percent of normal subjects but in 24 percent of disturbed children, 42 percent of psychiatric patients, and 52 percent of schizophrenics. In the 1970s, however, the mauve factor's identity was determined to be OHHPL (hydroxyhemoppyrrolin-2-one), not kryptopyrrole.[10]

Pyroluria is a genetic error that causes overproduction of OHHPL during the synthesis of hemoglobin, the iron-rich component of blood that carries oxygen to tissues. Both zinc and vitamin B_6 have a chemical affinity for OHHPL molecules. They bond to them and are excreted in the urine, thereby stripping the body of excess OHHPL, zinc, and B_6.

This creates problems because vitamin B_6 is an essential cofactor in the last step for producing the neurotransmitter serotonin. GABA (gamma-amino butyric acid), an amino acid and neurotransmitter equally vital for mental health, is also zinc dependent. Vitamin B_6 is a part of more than two thousand enzymes involved in digestion and metabolism, and zinc is required for the functioning of sixty enzymes and amino acid use.[11] Both aid digestion, which nourishes the brain and promotes health.

Pyroluria leaves people unable to cope with stress. Symptoms include severe mood swings, high anxiety, depression, episodic rage, little or no dream recall, reading disorders, and underachievement. Testing can be done through urine samples.[12] Treatment simply involves supplementing with higher-than-normal levels of zinc and vitamin B_6 to compensate for the loss.

Over- and Undermethylation

Methylation is a critical biochemical process (one of the detoxification pathways) that happens over a billion times a second in your body. It is rapidly becoming a hot topic because scientists have learned that impaired methylation contributes to cardiovascular disease, arthritis, and aging, and that it may be the genesis of cancer.[13]

Genes consist of double strands of DNA (deoxyribonucleic acid) that carry genetic information. Each cell in the body has two copies of every gene, one copy coming from our mother and one from our father (except those determining sex). Each gene has instructions for making a single protein or enzyme.[14]

Genes that program your physical appearance are fixed, but the scientific field of nutrigenomics (how genes and nutrition interact) has shown that those directing other biochemical processes in the body are always responding to foods you eat, to your emotions, to stress, and to the microenvironment within your cells.[15] Complex regulatory proteins control whether these genes are expressed or not expressed, whether they are turned "on" or "off."

One of these controls is SAMe (S-adenosyl-L-methionine), a compound in each cell assembled from an amino acid, methionine, and adenosine triphosphate (ATP, a molecule that provides energy to cells). SAMe delivers methyl groups (one carbon atom and three hydrogen atoms) that are added to or subtracted from other molecules to prompt actions at the cellular level—everything from immune function to cellular growth and repair.[16]

For example, noradrenaline is produced in the brain to keep you feeling happy. If you are in danger, the body adds a methyl group to noradrenaline to make adrenaline, giving you a burst of energy leading to the "fight or flight" response. When the emergency is over, the methyl group is taken away.[17]

The number and placement of methyl groups by enzymes provides a signal, a "tag" indicating which genes should be turned off or on. A failure in tagging, abnormal placement of tags due to aging (connected to lupus), and abnormal increases or decreases in tags (found with cancers), plus brain malfunctions are just a few of the areas now being studied.[18]

In late 2005, 450 scientists gathered in Durham, North Carolina, to discuss how methyl groups control genes and the impact of environmental toxins on methylation. Researchers are discovering that changes occurring in embryonic or fetal development from environmental assailants may contribute to an adult's susceptibility to obesity, heart disease, diabetes, and other conditions. The good news from the conference was that studies in pregnant mice showed that nutritional supplements B_{12}, folic acid, choline, and betaine from sugar beets can impact methylation and alter gene function, meaning the damage may be reversible through nutrition.[19]

The supplement SAMe has long been used in Europe as an antidepressant but was not available in this country until the late 1990s. By 2002, the U.S. government issued results of a study stating that SAMe was not only safe, it was *as effective as prescription antidepressants for depression*, and it was as effective as nonsteroidal anti-inflammatory drugs for joint and muscle pain, plus it improved liver function.[20] As an antioxidant with a key role in methylation, SAMe has a unique power to reverse damage caused by free radicals.

Many clinicians did not recommend SAMe to patients because it sometimes triggered anxiety or mania. Since they did not know how to differentiate between patients who overmethylate or undermethylate, it was simply ruled out. Pfeiffer Treatment Center, however, highly recommends SAMe, but only for patients who undermethylate as a result of deficient methylation systems.

Methylation can be determined by measuring imbalances of histamine (a product of metabolism that functions as a neurotransmitter, although best known for inducing allergies). In the 1970s, Dr. Pfeiffer discovered that nearly two-thirds of schizophrenics had histamine imbalances and he found that he could alleviate schizophrenic symptoms by giving supplements that normalized histamine levels. Because methyl groups and histamine are ubiquitous in the body and compete with each other, histamine levels thus became a good "marker" for measuring methylation. People with high histamine are undermethylated; those low in histamine are overmethylated.[21]

Undermethylation causes low levels of serotonin, dopamine, and norepinephrine with elevated histamine and excessive levels of folic acid. Symptoms include seasonal allergies, obsessive-compulsive tendencies, perfectionism, competitiveness, high libido, and sparse body hair. Pfeiffer Treatment Center recommends avoiding folic acid supplements and prescribes calcium (to help bring down a patient's histamine level), magnesium, zinc, vitamin B_6, manganese, inositol, vitamins C and E, omega-3 fatty acids, and the amino acid methionine or SAMe.

Methionine is a sulfur-containing amino acid that helps in detoxification and lowers levels of histamine. It also helps in the breakdown of fats and is a powerful antioxidant that protects against destructive free radicals. Plentiful in most protein sources—meats, dairy products, eggs, beans, and soy—it is also found in garlic, onions, and seeds. People may become deficient in methionine from not enough dietary protein or from the inability to digest and metabolize protein foods properly.

Some individuals lack the ability to convert methionine into SAMe and need to use supplements. Both methionine and supplemental SAMe directly introduce new methyl groups into the body, but if inadequate conversion is suspected, SAMe should be taken. Trimethylglycine (TMG), a less expensive supplement made from beets,[22] uses a secondary biochemical pathway, converting the small amount of homocysteine in the cycle to methionine, then SAMe.

Overmethylation causes elevated levels of dopamine, norepinephrine, and serotonin, and low levels of histamine. The incidence of overmethylation among one thousand five hundred people with bipolar disorder treated at Pfeiffer Treatment Center is about 18 percent.[23] Symptoms include numerous chemical and food sensitivities, high anxiety, low libido, obsessions but not compulsions, a tendency toward paranoia, auditory hallucinations, underachievement, "nervous" legs, and grandiosity. Natural supplements prescribed to reduce methyl levels include folic acid, vitamin B_{12} (sometimes administered by injection), niacin, choline, manganese, zinc, supportive vitamins C and E, and omega-3 fatty acids in fish oils. People who overmethylate should avoid taking supplements of methionine, SAMe, inositol, or TMG.

According to Dr. Walsh, insufficient folic acid (now also called vitamin B_9) is a major cause of overmethylation. A study of patients with megaloblastic anemia demonstrated that those with clear folate deficiencies (but adequate vitamin B_{12}) showed an incidence of mood disturbances exceeding 50 percent.[24] Derived from the term *foliage*, folate is found in green leafy vegetables, such as broccoli, spinach, and lettuces, as well as in beans and rice. People suffering from celiac disease, irritable bowel syndrome, Crohn's disease, or other ailments that interfere with food absorption often have a deficiency in folic acid.

Metal Metabolism

Dr. Walsh has found that two-thirds of people with behavior disorders, including those with hormonal depression and ADHD, have problems metabolizing trace metals. The genetic inability to metabolize copper, zinc, manganese, and other trace metals in the body is caused by improper functioning of metallothionein—a small protein, synthesized in the liver and kidney in response to the presence of metal ions. Such patients have a deficiency of zinc, manganese, vitamin B_6, and the amino acids cysteine and serine. They also show excessive levels of copper, lead, and cadmium.[25]

Because there is no commercial test to measure metallothionein, Pfeiffer Treatment Center uses blood-level ratios of zinc, copper, and ceruloplasmin as indicators of a malfunction in metal metabolism. Such patients must avoid high copper found in shellfish, chocolate, and carob, as well as enriched foods and other copper-containing substances. Drinking bottled water is recommended, since acidic tap water may leach the mineral from copper piping.

In addition to brain disorders, symptoms of elevated copper include hormonal imbalances and intolerance to estrogen. Treatment involves supplementing where there are deficiencies of zinc, manganese, cysteine, serine, and vitamin B_6 to stimulate metallothionein production.

Celiac Disease

Since my early twenties, I was able to connect feeling "down" to eating too many carbohydrates. In 2002, having solved the symptoms of mania and depression, I consulted Dr. O'Connor again to work on improving my flawed digestion. Stool sample analysis revealed a complete absence in my gut of acidophilus, one of the usually plentiful, beneficial bacteria. Although antibiotics are known to kill off acidophilus, I had not taken any in five years. Based on an educated hunch, Dr. O'Connor ordered a gluten antibody blood test. Two days later, she called to say that I had celiac disease.

Celiac disease (also called celiac sprue) is a genetically based allergic reaction to a protein called gluten, which is found in nearly all grains except rice. The disease typically causes diarrhea, gas, cramping, and weight loss, or it might show up as joint pain, fatigue, or a skin rash. I had no digestive symptoms.

It is not uncommon to have celiac disease many years before it is diagnosed. A 2003 survey of five thousand members of the Canadian Celiac Association showed the average age of those with the illness was fifty-five, and the average age at diagnosis was forty-five. Most diagnoses came in response to symptoms ranging from abdominal pain and diarrhea to fatigue or weight loss.[26] It appears possible that celiac genes might be turned off in our youth and get turned on as we age.

It is believed that when a person has celiac disease, his immune system reacts to gluten as foreign. Human leukocyte antigen (HLA) molecules, found on the surface of cells and involved in immune regulation, bind to small fragments of peptides (amino acids), bacteria, or viruses and "present" these to T-cells patrolling the body to ward off intruders. When a T-cell concludes that something is foreign, it issues an alarm and the immune system sends an army of antibodies to eliminate the intruders. Over time, this repeated immune response to gluten in the small intestine results in a flattening of the villi—billions of hairlike projections lining the gut that absorb nutrients—resulting in malabsorption of nutrients, which is also a hallmark of mental illness.

Although celiac-related HLA markers can be tested for, there are numerous variants of the HLA molecule and it is not completely understood why only some react to gluten. Thus, their presence does not predict whether or not celiac disease will develop. About 25–30 percent of people of European extraction have celiac-related HLA markers—the same ones found in 95 percent of all celiac sufferers. Since the disease affects only 1 out of 250 people in Europe and the United States (0.4%), what causes this gene to be turned on has yet to be determined.[27]

The National Institutes of Health estimate that 3 million Americans may suffer from celiac disease. The family incidence is roughly 10 percent among first-degree relatives. Among identical twins, it is 70 percent, indicating that there are both genetic and nongenetic factors, such as viruses or stress triggers, involved.

Your genes need not sentence you to a life of mental illness. They can be turned on or off by foods, emotions, stress, hormones, and environmental factors that are under your control. While identifying genetic problems was an integral part of my healing, in many cases it is unnecessary. As you will see from the subsequent stories, most people notice mental improvements as soon as they start taking supplements that provide the raw materials required by the body to perform an array of unseen, vital internal functions.

CHAPTER 2

Brain Basics: Vitamins, Minerals, and Good Fats

Kassidi Bishop was a clearheaded kid, who knew at an early age precisely what she wanted to do in life and was well on her way. The five-foot-eleven blonde had become such an outstanding basketball player that by her freshman year in high school she had received upward of four hundred college recruiting letters.

In April, a few days before her sixteenth birthday, Kassidi came down with chicken pox. Within three weeks, she was experiencing profound mood swings and made her first suicide attempt in June. Kassidi's life became a rapid, descending spiral, from an honors student in three subjects to a high school dropout. "I didn't understand why I was feeling the way I was. I was angry at basketball, angry with my family, and I didn't know what I wanted to do anymore. Things just went downhill," she recalls.

Finally diagnosed with clinical depression, Kassidi was put on medication, although she doesn't remember which one because thirteen different drugs were prescribed during the course of her illness. "Of course, if you put bipolar [people] on depression medications, it spikes them into mania," she says, "which we found out the hard way."

Coached to success in basketball by her father and always close to both her parents, the bipolar Kassidi ran away from home to live with an abusive boyfriend. Physically violent and a "control freak," the boyfriend installed a deadbolt lock on the outside of their apartment door so he could lock her in when he left. "I'd sit in a depression for two weeks and not change my clothes," Kassidi says. When manic, she would wash each load of laundry four or five times to be sure it was clean. Or, deciding to cook dinner, she would bake a turkey, then fix spaghetti, cooking four to six meals in one day. "It was just bizarre. I look back on it now and I just roll my eyes," she says.

Between the age of sixteen and eighteen, Kassidi made three suicide attempts and began to "self-medicate very heavily with alcohol." When her boyfriend's violence escalated to daily beatings and he nearly severed the spinal cord in her neck, the police were called, Kassidi was hospitalized, and the relationship ended.

"I was supposed to be the next Miss Basketball Colorado," says Kassidi. It was extremely difficult to go from being a high-profile, all-American athlete before her illness to hearing the media ask: Where is Kassidi Bishop? What's wrong with her?

"There was always this string of sanity holding me to the direction I should be following, to the clear path. I hoped if I got back into school and basketball, things would be better." Because of her stellar reputation on the hardwood, offers still kept coming.

"In the fall of 1995, I was contacted by a coach in Odessa, Texas, who said if I got my GED [General Educational Development test that shows high school equivalency], they would give me a scholarship in January of 1996." Kassidi obtained her GED, enrolled in Odessa College, and maintained close to a 3.9 grade point average. Things were looking up.

"Two and a half weeks before the end of the semester, for what reason I have no idea, I packed a bag, jumped on a Greyhound bus, and came home. I didn't notify the school, my coach, nothing, and, obviously, I failed." It was a pattern that continued for six terms.

"In fall of 1997, I got an offer to come play college basketball in California. All the while, I'm still up and down on medications and self-medicating, but my reputation allowed me another opportunity." Again, she did well at first before things once again fell apart.

There was a silver lining to her California sojourn, however.

A doctor, John Nasse, in the town of Ojai, made a "real connection" with the desperate young woman. "I really despised going to doctors," Kassidi explains. "They would put me on medication, I'd feel better for about two weeks, and then the side effects would start kicking in," she explains. "I would react to the side effects, come off my medications, and spin off in the wrong direction. Then the doctors would ask me, 'What are you feeling?' I just got *tired* of it, repeating my story over and over, with no one finding a solution. Instead of analyzing what I was thinking, I just wanted someone to *help* me.

"Dr. Nasse started me on lithium and Wellbutrin. At the same time, he was researching studies, looking at vitamins and nutrients that help stop the cravings and reverse the effects of alcoholism. He talked to me about my diet, cutting down on sugar, not drinking milk. He started to nudge me into natural, alternative treatment while I was taking medications."

She hated the drugs. Kassidi nearly blacked out during practice from the effects of lithium during strenuous exercise, her hair came out in clumps, and her eyesight deteriorated. "With lithium, it's pretty darn difficult to catch a basketball when your hands are shaking. I had tremors so bad I couldn't hold a pen, literally. My performance was altered due to the side effects, but I gutted it out. There was nothing that would stop me from succeeding." Kassidi continued taking the drugs because of her trust in Dr. Nasse. Gradually, her moods stabilized.

Having failed both semesters in California, she returned home again. In the spring of 1998, "I said, 'Daddy, I want to play basketball,' and he kind of looked at me like, right, I've heard this one before," she recounts with a laugh. He offered her a deal: If she would finish one full year of classes, he would talk about it.

More stable at this point, Kassidi passed all her classes during both fall and spring semesters, so her father began helping her find a scholarship and an opportunity to play. NCAA rules state that athletes have only five years to complete four years of college, and the clock starts once they enter any college, regardless of whether they play a sport or not. Since Kassidi had enrolled in college in January 1996 and this was 1999, she only had two years to finish. "The NCAA rules also say if you receive a GED, you must obtain an associate's degree before you're eligible to transfer to a Division I or Division II university to compete." Kassidi needed to find a junior college where she could get an associate's degree in one year.

A coach from Sheridan College in Wyoming gave her a scholarship and became her advisor, telling Kassidi she needed sixteen class hours the first semester and sixteen the second to obtain her degree. "I enrolled, moved up to Sheridan," Kassidi says, "and averaged roughly seventeen points a game that first semester. I was playing extremely well."

Meanwhile, her mother was also diagnosed as bipolar. Although Kassidi's genetic tendency was probably always present, "The doctors believe that the chicken pox virus attacked the serotonin levels of my brain, triggering that first bipolar episode."

Both women suffered severe side effects from the psychiatric drugs, so Kassidi's father began researching alternative treatments. Through the Internet, he found Truehope, a fledgling Canadian nonprofit organization that was conducting a clinical study of its new all-natural vitamin/mineral/amino acid supplement, EMPowerplus.[1] The researchers were extremely interested in having Kassidi join the study, since most other participants were overweight, institutionalized patients not in good health. "They were curious how my body would react because I had very low body fat, a high metabolism, and was athletic."

Her father asked what she thought of trying the supplement. Kassidi was "a little nervous. After finally getting the opportunity to play, I'm doing well, and I'm passing my classes, and stabilized. Why do I want to throw a wrench in it and have everything blow up again?" But she says, "I thought, 'Well, I have bad side effects, and there's always going to be a pharmaceutical company out there, so if this natural treatment doesn't work, I'll just go back on the drugs.'"

The plan was for her to stay on both her prior medications and take

EMPowerplus for eight weeks, then taper off the drugs. "Within three days of starting the supplement, I called my dad and said, 'Something's wrong. I can't see. My eyes are open and it's black and I have the worst headache.'" Kassidi thought she was dying or had a brain tumor.

Her father called Truehope. A telephone conference call was hastily arranged with Kassidi in Wyoming, her internist in Colorado, Dr. Nasse in California, and the Canadian doctors. They concluded that her body chemistry had normalized so quickly from the supplement that she was in the midst of a toxic reaction to lithium. They told her to stop taking the drug immediately.

"I just took a leap of faith and prayed that nothing was going to go wrong," she says. Three days later, her vision was normal and "My thinking was so incredibly clear and sharp, more than it had ever been. The medications numb your emotions and your thinking is cloudy. On the minerals, I had never felt that clear-minded since being diagnosed. It was truly amazing.

"I was extremely fortunate. I almost think it was God's work, because I finished up my semester." A clear mind became even more essential when Kassidi discovered that her coach had made a rather large miscalculation: The athlete needed 26 class hours the second semester—not 16, as she had been told—in order to obtain her associate's degree within the mandated time frame. Determined and feeling great, she obtained special permission to continue at Sheridan College and take online classes too, committing to 26½ hours for the spring semester.

In a practice after Christmas, Kassidi went up for a jump shot, jumped, and broke her right ankle. She was utterly despondent. "I finally have the opportunity. I'm playing great. I'm stabilized. I break my ankle. I need to get recruited to go to Division I, and now I'm not going to play the second half of the season."

While the broken ankle healed, she had extra time to study. Kassidi passed all her classes. "I was ecstatic. It was a very long road. My family didn't get to see me graduate from high school, so to see me graduate with an associate's degree was quite extraordinary. It was very joyful."

Recruited by the University of Louisville in Kentucky, she had one year of school left, but only a half-season to play. "I appealed to the NCAA, asking for my eligibility back. My argument was that they grant eligibility back all the time to people with a torn knee or who are hospitalized with diabetes. My mental illness was no different." In December 2000, the NCAA ruled for the first time in history to grant eligibility based on a mental illness.

The Associated Press released Kassidi's story. It was carried all over the United States and Europe. ESPN's show *Outside the Lines* did an entire thirty-minute segment on the athlete that aired New Year's Eve. Truehope in Canada, the university's athletic department, and Kassidi were inundated with calls for months. The spotlight had returned, but this time the focus was different.

"All I ever hoped for when I was very, very sick was to hear someone speak out where I could say, 'Ah, that's how I feel.' And hear that person saying it's going to be okay. But there was no one. So, I thought, this is my opportunity to help people struggling who face those same demons inside on a day-in, day-out basis. Maybe when they've lost all hope, maybe they'd hear my story or read something about me and think, maybe it will be okay, and just that glimpse of light will keep them from committing suicide."

Months later, Kassidi was distressed to learn that Truehope did not *require* physician supervision of patients transitioning from psychiatric drugs to the natural supplement. Since her story, and her name, were prompting thousands to take EMPowerplus, "that was extremely worrisome to me. That's one of the quickest ways to have someone get into trouble or commit suicide. You can't just have them stop their medication."

Her father was also concerned, but for a different reason. The Canadian Ministry of Health was threatening to classify the all-natural supplement as a drug simply because it was so effective. The economic ramifications of this change would in effect remove it from the market, to the joy of the pharmaceutical companies. To assure his daughter and wife a continued supply, Kassidi's father worked with a laboratory in Oklahoma to create a similar, less expensive supplement—named Quiet Mind—and ordered a ten-year supply. It is the only supplement Kassidi still takes regularly, and the family now sells it.[2]

What else does Kassidi do to maintain mental stability? "I think it's important for people with mental illness to be active, get exercise, get adequate sleep, and eat right. If I don't get at least eight hours' sleep a night, I can feel it the next day." She does not drink soda or eat anything containing aspartame (NutraSweet®, Equal®, and Spoonful®); does not consume sports drinks because of their high sugar levels; and avoids sugars, caffeine, flour, and bread.

With a political science degree from the University of Louisville, Kassidi has applied to law school, intent on becoming a sports agent. "I read somewhere that perhaps as many as 20 percent of athletes and entertainers are bipolar. So, who would be a better agent for them than someone who's been there?"

The Brain's Need for Vitamins, Minerals, and Good Fats

If a simple vitamin/mineral/amino acid supplement can compensate for inherited tendencies, aid recovery after a viral attack, and repair a malfunctioning brain, why haven't you heard about these miraculous natural compounds? Because, until recently, supplement manufacturers were prevented from making health claims for their products, and there are slim profits from natural supplements compared to patented drugs. However, here is a brief look at some of the vitamins, minerals, and healthy fats the body *must have* to run right.

Eight B-vitamins are also called coenzymes because they assist enzymes that trigger millions of vital biochemical reactions in the body (more on this in chapter 5). All B-vitamins are water-soluble, meaning the body cannot store any excess, so they have to be replaced continually through diet or supplements. Also referred to as the B-complex vitamins, they act synergistically: They are more potent when taken together and in balance. Each has a numerical designation, one or more scientific names, and collectively they have a tremendous beneficial impact on the brain.

Vitamin B$_1$, Thiamine, acts as a coenzyme in the conversion of glucose (blood sugar)—the brain's primary fuel—into energy. Used for the production of an important neurotransmitter, acetylcholine, thiamine is linked with improving the ability to learn. High sugar or alcohol consumption can deplete supplies of thiamine. The first symptoms of a deficiency are fatigue, irritability, emotional instability, and poor concentration. Chronic mild deficiency may cause people to hear voices or have nightmares. Psychosis can result from a severe deficiency.[3]

Vitamin B$_2$, Riboflavin, is America's most commonly deficient vitamin. It works to energize and clean cells, acting as an antioxidant against free radicals, and it works with other substances to break down carbohydrates, fats, and proteins. Physical symptoms of B$_2$ deficiency are fatigue, cracks or sores in the corners of the mouth, vision problems, and stunted growth in children. Mental symptoms are forgetfulness, lack of concentration, and mild confusion.[4]

Vitamin B$_3$, Niacin, is a precursor to two coenzymes needed for brain metabolism. It is used in the formation of key neurotransmitters—serotonin, histamine, and acetylcholine—as well as the regulation of dopamine and copper levels.[5] Excessive intake of sugar, starches, and certain antibiotics can exhaust the body's supply of niacin. Available from protein foods, a deficiency causes disturbed behavior, irritability, and in some people may promote cravings for alcohol, tobacco, or addictive substances.

Vitamin B$_5$, Pantothenic Acid, plays a vital role in the digestion of carbohydrates, fats, and proteins. Since it is widely available in foods, deficiencies were thought to be rare. However, 33 percent of the vitamin in meat is lost during cooking, 50 percent in wheat is lost during the processing of flour, and 33 percent can be lost by baking or cooking with dry heat, vinegars (acids), or baking soda (alkali). Shortages of B$_5$ may cause low levels of hydrochloric acid in the stomach and poor digestion; low blood sugar and depression; and quarrelsome, hot-tempered behavior, or insomnia.[6]

Vitamin B$_6$, Pyridoxine, is one of the most vital vitamins for brain health. It is responsible for production of the neurotransmitter GABA and supports formation of dopamine, norepinephrine, and acetylcholine. Vitamin B$_6$ supplements are used to treat depression, bipolar disorder, schizophrenia, autism, epilepsy, hyperactivity, and anxiety. Care must be used when taking large doses of B$_6$ for a prolonged period, however. Too much B$_6$ can cause an imbalance of other B-vitamins, and without adequate zinc, may cause nerve damage, signaled by numbness and tingling in fingers and toes.[7]

Vitamin B$_9$, Folic Acid or **Folate,** is found in green leafy vegetables (as well as in beans and rice). It is essential to mental health because it works with vitamins B$_{12}$ and C in the breakdown and metabolism of proteins. Frequently deficient in the diet, low levels are also found where illnesses (such as celiac disease) or drugs interfere with food absorption, or with use of oral contraceptives, sulfa drugs, the anticonvulsant Dilantin, barbiturates, estrogen, or alcohol.

Vitamin B$_{12}$, Cobalamin, is needed only in minute amounts, but adequate supplies are absolutely vital to the central nervous system. Vitamin B$_{12}$ allows for normal metabolism of protein, fat, and carbohydrates. Deficiencies are common even when blood levels measure normal, due to a molecule transport defect. Low levels cause depression, confusion, memory gaps, anxiety, and seizures. Small doses with several meals are better absorbed than a large dose, but the vitamin is poorly absorbed in the stomach unless the intrinsic factor (a small gastric-secreted protein) is present. To bypass the gut, sublingual (under the tongue) lozenges or injections are often prescribed for severe shortages. For the body to use vitamin B$_{12}$, there must also be adequate calcium, iron, and vitamins B$_6$ and B$_9$.[8] Vegans or vegetarians often have diets low in B$_{12}$ but high in folic acid, an imbalance that can mask a B$_{12}$ deficiency. In bipolar patients, monitoring is important because high supplementation of B$_{12}$ may trigger mania.

Biotin, part of the B-complex vitamins, works in tandem with B$_2$,

B$_5$, B$_6$, and B$_9$ and plays a role in fat metabolism. Made by intestinal bacteria, it helps stabilize blood sugar levels and mood.[9]

Vitamin A (including **Carotenes**) occurs naturally in two forms. Preformed A is in animal tissues, such as fish liver oil and all meats, and in milk, cheese, butter, and eggs. Beta-carotene, the "precursor" form, comes from dark green, yellow, and deep orange fruits and vegetables and must be converted to vitamin A by the body before it can be used. Vitamin A enables the body to utilize vitamins B, C, E, and K, promoting growth and repair of tissues. An antioxidant, it protects neurotransmitter receptors and enhances immune function. Chronic stress causes depletion of vitamin A, and low levels are common among depressed patients.[10]

Vitamin C, Ascorbic Acid, assists in the formation of the neurotransmitters norepinephrine and serotonin. In high doses, it may act as a natural tranquilizer or antipsychotic, since it fits into dopamine receptor sites. Vitamin C is essential to adrenal function, elimination of toxins, including heavy metals, and resistance to stress. It also promotes wound healing, maintenance of collagen, cholesterol regulation, the disabling of viruses and infections, and it aids in the metabolism of other vitamins. The ability to absorb vitamin C is impaired by smoking, digestive disorders, stress, aging, inflammation, aspirin, and high fever. Depression is the first clinical symptom of low vitamin C.[11]

Vitamin D comes from food or exposure to sunlight. The sun's ultraviolet rays activate your cholesterol, converting it to vitamin D. It takes only fifteen minutes of sun exposure on the face and arms three times a week for the body to make what it needs. Sunscreens of 8 or above, however, block this process. Although most people know that vitamin D is necessary for the formation of strong bones and teeth (which is why it is added to milk), most are unaware that it contributes to mental health through its role in thyroid production.

Deficiencies of vitamin D are associated with hypothyroidism, seasonal affective disorder (SAD), anxiety, suicide, insomnia, substance abuse, and convulsions. Taking cholesterol-lowering drugs, antacids, mineral oil, and steroids can interfere with absorption. Vitamin D is fat-soluble, meaning the body does store it. Thus, excesses from too much supplementation—but not from sun exposure—can be toxic. Recommended intake is 400 IU in summer and 800 IU in winter. Natural dietary D_3 comes from fish liver oils, liver, and eggs. Vitamin D_2 is a synthetic form used for food fortification.[12]

Vitamin E, Tocopherol, an antioxidant, plays a major role in cellular health, protecting DNA, cell membranes, and enzymes from free radical damage. It enhances brain circulation, increases concentration and memory, and lifts mild depression. One collaborative study at major medical centers across the U.S. found that 2,000 mg daily delayed the progression of Alzheimer's memory loss by seven months.[13] Also fat-soluble, vitamin E can be safely ingested in daily doses of 400 to 600 IU.

Minerals and the Brain

Boron is a trace mineral needed in minuscule amounts but with a significant role in nerve signal transmission, enhancing alertness. Found in apples, carrots, grapes, leafy vegetables, nuts, pears, and grains, but deficient in junk-food diets, it is needed for proper absorption of vitamin D, calcium, and magnesium.

Calcium is the most abundant mineral in the body, with 99 percent found in bones and teeth. Calcium levels in bones fluctuate, however, depending on the body's calcium needs for other processes. If there is not enough in the diet, calcium is withdrawn from bone reserves to maintain the cardiovascular system, to assist with blood clotting, and to serve as a messenger from cell surfaces to the interior. Calcium affects the neurotransmitters serotonin, acetylcholine, and norepinephrine; nerve transmission; use of phosphorus and magnesium; and aids in B_{12} utilization. It helps control histamine levels that, when elevated, cause phobias, compulsions, depression, and psychosis. Calcium absorption is inefficient, so it is best to take small doses several times a day and before bedtime (as it aids deep, restful sleep).[14]

Chromium acts as a transporter of the amino acid tryptophan across the blood-brain barrier, where it is converted to the feel-good neurotransmitter serotonin. An essential trace element, needed for metabolism and enzyme activity, it also regulates insulin, making chromium one of the first nutrients I recommend for people with mood swings due to low blood sugar or diabetes.[15]

Copper is a conductor of electricity that helps regulate neurotransmitter levels and maintain myelin, the insulating sheath surrounding nerve cells. Copper and zinc help keep each other in balance and should be in a ratio of roughly 1:10.[16] According to Pfeiffer Treatment Center, low levels of copper cause poor concentration, confrontational behavior, fascination with fire, cruelty, sleep disorders, numbness and tingling in extremities, and anorexia. Elevated levels of copper cause Jekyll-Hyde behavior, episodic violence, poor stress control, and academic underachievement. Manganese and zinc supplements can be used to bring down high levels of copper.[17]

Iodine is used by thyroid hormones that control the body's energy production and metabolic rate. In brain cells, thyroid hormones enable production and function of neurotransmitters. Iodine is so vital to health that the U.S. government mandated that table salt be iodized fifty years ago to prevent goiters and hypothyroidism. Classic symptoms of low iodine (or thyroid) are depression, weight gain, low energy, and cold feet or hands.

Iron, used for production of red blood corpuscles, helps transport oxygen throughout the body, including the brain. An iron deficiency is one of the most common nutritional deficiencies in children—a Johns Hopkins University study published by *Lancet* in 1996 showed a direct relationship between increases in blood iron levels and the ability to learn.[18] Copper, cobalt, manganese, and vitamin C are all necessary for assimilation of iron. In turn, adequate iron is essential for use of the vital B-vitamins. Too much iron, however, generates free radicals and disease. Since balance is critical, and there are genetic conditions that cause iron overload, blood levels should *always* be measured before taking any supplemental iron, in vitamins or fortified foods.

Magnesium contributes to emotional balance by aiding the release and uptake of serotonin and is a cofactor in more than 250 enzymatic reactions (more on enzymes in chapter 5).[19] When we feel stressed, the body uses more. Thus, in our overstressed culture, most people run low. Attention deficit hyperactivity disorder, delinquency, and childhood depression are all associated with magnesium deficiency.[20] Because magnesium and calcium compete for the same absorption sites, supplements with 1,000 mg of calcium and 500 mg of magnesium are customary, although a 1:1 ratio often boosts energy and healing.

Manganese is used in the regulation of neurotransmitters and in glucose metabolism, protein digestion, and cholesterol and fatty acid synthesis. It is a cofactor for use of vitamins B_1, C, and E, and aids in detoxification and hormone functions.[21]

Molybdenum is a trace mineral required by enzymes for detoxification, including heavy metals (see chapter 6). It is found in practically all plant and animal tissues, and only recently have deficiencies been identified, due to food processing, refining, or an accumulation of sulfite preservatives in foods and drugs.

Potassium, with sodium, helps regulate water balance in the body. It is every element's helper: working with phosphorus to send oxygen to the brain; with calcium to regulate neuromuscular activity; and assisting in conversion of the brain's primary fuel, glucose. Potassium activates enzymes and is needed for protein and carbohydrate use. Essential for transmission of nerve impulses to the brain, it helps control mood swings. Low supplies can result from excessive consumption of alcohol, coffee, refined sugar, diuretics, laxatives, and cortisone; from digestive diseases; or from not eating enough fruits and vegetables.[22]

Selenium has become a rising nutrient star since researchers discovered that a deficiency allows a normally benign virus, coxsackievirus, to mutate into a vicious form, and that inadequate levels in mice allow a mild influenza virus to become virulent.[23] Three separate studies have connected selenium deficiencies in the brain with increased depression, anxiety, hostility, or confusion. A potent antioxidant, selenium neutralizes damaging free radicals, helps make active thyroid hormone available, and assists in removing toxins from the body, protecting against a buildup that can disrupt brain function.

Zinc is one of the minerals most vital to brain health. Used for neurotransmitter synthesis, it is an element in more than sixty enzymes involved in digestion and metabolism. It is a component of insulin and is necessary for growth and repair of tissue. Zinc helps control copper levels, since the two elements compete for absorption sites in the small intestine. Zinc deficiencies are known to cause depression, violence, dyslexia, anorexia, and nerve damage.[24]

Essential Fatty Acids

The brain is 60 percent fat by weight and requires ongoing supplies of essential fatty acids (EFAs) to function. The body cannot manufacture them, so they must come from diet, and they are the basic ingredient of nerve cells, cellular membranes, and prostaglandins (hormonelike molecules) throughout the body.

What we eat is directly integrated into cell membranes, becoming the "envelope" protecting the cell and through which cells interact. The type of fat we eat impacts both form and function. Large quantities of saturated fats—those solid at room temperature—cause the nerve cell membranes to become rigid. If we eat mostly polyunsaturated fats (including omega-3 fatty acids)—which are liquid at room temperature—the membranes become fluid and flexible, helping stabilize cellular communication.

In recent research by Harvard psychiatry professor Perry F. Renshaw, magnetic resonance imaging found that depressed people's brains had stiffer cell membranes. He drew the analogy that cell membranes were like an ocean, with neurotransmitter receptors the floating buoys. Rigid membranes mean the receptors can't float as freely, reducing their responsiveness.[25]

Of eight EFAs, there are two main groups, omega-3s and omega-6s. Omega-3s control the immune response, prevent blood stickiness, reduce inflammation, and are considered "good." Omega-6s, although essential to stimulating immune response and for adequate blood clotting, become "bad" in excess, making the blood too thick and causing high levels of inflammation.

EFAs regulate and enhance mood, sharpen memory, and aid concentration and learning. The secret to mental and physical health, however, lies in the *balance* of omega-6s and -3s. Americans regularly consume large amounts of omega-6s in meats, chicken, cheese, eggs, nuts, and vegetable oils. They eat far fewer omega-3s, found primarily in cold-water seafood, flaxseed, marine vegetation, green leafy land vegetables, and beans. A healthy balance of omega-6s to omega-3s is believed to be between 6:1 and 1:1. By some estimates Americans consume a 20:1 ratio, resulting in an inflammatory "cascade" that leads to arthritis, heart disease, tumor development, and brain disorders.

Harvard researcher Andrew Stoll, M.D., conducted clinical trials using ten grams of omega-3 fish oils daily to successfully end bipolar symptoms, described in his book *The Omega-3 Connection*.[26] There are three main types of omega-3 fats: eicosapentaenoic acid (EPA), docosahexaenoic acid (DHA), and alpha-linolenic acid (ALA). EPA and DHA are found mostly in seafood. ALA comes from plants, like flaxseeds, walnuts, and tofu.

According to Dr. Stoll, EPA is the active anti-inflammatory omega-3 and the most mood-promoting agent in fish oil. The fish oil supplements Stoll went on to create, Omega Brite brand, have seven times as much EPA as DHA in order to raise mood more quickly than conventional fish oils. Vegetarians may be tempted to substitute flaxseeds or flaxseed oil instead, but only a fraction of ALA (between 10 and 15 percent) is converted to the other more powerful omega-3s, so plant sources are not likely to provide adequate mood-altering benefits.[27]

EFAs require vitamins B_3, B_6, and C, along with the minerals magnesium and zinc, for use. Even with these cofactors present, however, the body's conversion of good fats can be blocked by intake of trans-fatty acids or hydrogenated oils, often found in baked goods. Since fats are highly perishable, hydrogenated oils (where an extra hydrogen ion is added) extend the shelf life of most commercial breads, crackers, and cookies carried by conventional grocery stores. Rarely are these altered fats used in products carried in health food stores, but do read labels because unhealthy fried foods are staples of both types of stores.

Avoid anything fried, regardless of the type of oil used, because high heat uses up the antioxidants in oil and produces free radicals that start chain reactions, creating trans fats and, worse still, scores of unnatural, destructive chemicals that cause cells to degenerate over time.[28] For example, the California attorney general has filed a lawsuit to force makers of potato chips and french fries to warn consumers about a potential cancer-causing substance in their products. The chemical, acrylamide, is formed when any starchy foods is cooked at high heat.

Other factors that block the body's use of essential fatty acids are saturated animal fats, alcohol, chemical carcinogens, and alas, aging.

Taking a high-potency vitamin and mineral supplement along with filtered fish oils is an easy first step for people with depression or bipolar disorder toward making certain their brain has some of the basic elements needed for optimum performance.

CHAPTER 3

Ruling Out Hormone Imbalances, Diseases, and Medications

Stress at work was causing insomnia, so Joy began taking six to eight Tylenol PM pills a night, far more than the recommended dose. Because she had always been exceptionally healthy, she was unaccustomed to taking medicine of any kind and did not realize that you had to be careful, even with over-the-counter drugs. Within three weeks, she felt strangely hyper and made an appointment with a psychiatrist, who after a "ten-minute interview" diagnosed her as bipolar, prescribed lithium, and put her in the hospital. Although she clearly told him she was taking this sleep aid, neither knew that the ingredient in Tylenol PM that makes you sleepy, the antihistamine diphenhydramine, can cause restlessness, excitement, and hallucinations in high doses.

A blond-haired, blue-eyed, thirty-six-year old of Scots, Irish, and German descent, Joy was an avid athlete. Once a cheerleader in school, she ran track, canoed on the river, hiked in the mountains, and swam frequently in the ocean. The only pills she took before the Tylenol were an occasional aspirin or vitamin C tablet.

In the hospital, Joy's mania subsided immediately. Her doctor was a bit surprised, commenting that lithium usually took longer to act. Upon discharge, he arranged for thyroid testing every six months, because the drug can interfere with the gland's function. When Joy asked exactly how lithium worked, however, she was amazed when he and every other doctor responded, "We don't know."

Six months later, Joy was shopping at a home interior show with a relative when her right foot "did this strange cramp and pulled right up out of my shoe. I could not get my shoe back on and my foot would not come out of the cramp." When she mentioned it to the doctor, he said it was not related to the medication.

She gained weight, adding about twenty-five pounds over a two-year period.

Tired of continued stress at her accounting job, she quit, taking a new position at Sears. Soon, "I noticed my feet were burning and stinging, so I thought it was my shoes at first." She experimented, wearing different pairs, to no avail. Occasionally, "My feet would burn so bad at night that I would get up and either put them in real cold water or massage them."

Next, Joy started having pain in her right hip. "I remember repositioning myself at my desk at different angles and repositioning my leg. Nothing helped. I couldn't understand where this pain was coming from because I had always been extremely athletic. The last two years I worked, I propped my leg up on a trash can and I was in severe pain, eating four Tylenol and four aspirin at the same time." The hip remained cramped for seven years.

Making the rounds of doctors in an attempt to find answers, Joy says, "I tried everything in the book—physical therapy first and then a chiropractor told me if I just sat right and used the right posture and diet, he could help me. I tried meditating for the pain, but when you're working you can't just meditate while doing accounting at the same time." She switched to a total vegetarian diet and eliminated all dairy products, thinking her pain was being caused by a food allergy. She ordered mushrooms from California with special healing bacteria. None of it had an impact.

One day at her country farmhouse, she was prying something with a crowbar when a new symptom developed. Not immediately, but three days later, Joy awoke with "the most severe rolling muscle spasm charging down my back all the way to my lower right hip." The muscle remained cramped for two months. The only way she could sleep was arched backward in bed, surrounded by pillows.

Her husband took her to over ten different types of medical specialists, from a brain surgeon to a neurologist to an orthopedist. She had two MRIs, CAT scans, and dozens of x-rays that showed nothing wrong. All the doctors said there was nothing they could do. She would just have to learn to live in pain.

Several times she asked her psychiatrist if there could be any connection between the pains and lithium. He reassured her there was not. Whenever her thyroid was checked, he said the results were normal.

The now-constant muscle spasms and agony eventually were diagnosed as fibromyalgia. Symptoms are painful trigger points in muscles, accompanied by joint swelling, numbness or tingling sensations, sleep disorders, anxiety, and depression.

Joy could no longer work but could not get disability. "If you can't show what's causing your pain, they don't give you disability. I don't know of any cases of people with fibromyalgia who can get it, because nothing shows up on the MRIs." According to Joy, some doctors at that time thought depression caused fibromyalgia, "But I believe excruciating pain can bring on depression because it gradually takes away everything in your life."

After five years on lithium, Joy became bedridden. "I could no longer drive an automobile. I could not walk to my mailbox. I was just housebound. There were days where I actually crawled to the bathroom." Her weight dropped from 140 to 89 pounds.

Her husband of nineteen years left her. Joy attempted suicide three times. At first, she slashed her wrists, but not deep enough, and made another unsuccessful attempt by taking sixty lithium pills. Once she sat locked in her bedroom for three days with a gun, debating about shooting herself. "I wanted to live, but I wanted to escape the pain."

Finally, crying in bed one night, she said, "I'm going to read. I've got to research and try to find a way to help myself. None of these doctors can help me. If I'm going to get better, I'm going to have to help myself."

From *Harrison's Principles of Internal Medicine*, Joy learned that *fibro* means "connective tissue," the thin membrane that wraps around muscles. *Myalgia* means "muscle pain." "The peripheral nervous system runs through connective tissue and skin, so when the muscles cramp, they are clamping down on hundreds of nerves, which is why fibromyalgia pain is so extreme," she explains.

The same month her husband left, a miracle occurred. A stranger walked into the shop where Joy's son worked as the sales manager and mentioned that he knew something to relieve chronic pain—magnets. Her son told her, but Joy was skeptical. Still, she called a listing for medical magnets in the Yellow Pages. She spoke with a young woman who had suffered a broken back, arm, and neck when an overhead air conditioner had fallen on her at work, leaving her suffering for years until a scientist told her about using magnets.

Blood contains iron that functions as a carrier of oxygen and carbon dioxide. Magnetism increases the electrical conductivity of the blood. As blood circulates, magnetized iron is able to transport more oxygen to cell tissue and remove more carbon dioxide waste. When a magnetic flux passes through tissue, a secondary current is created in cells, activating cell metabolism, causing muscle spasms to decrease, lessening inflammation, and aiding cell regeneration. The negative pole energies of magnetism also interfere with the nerve cell's ability to send pain impulses to the brain.[1]

Joy ordered a magnetic mattress pad from Norso Biomagnetics in High Point, North Carolina. After just two weeks of sleeping on the pad, she was able to walk again and do all her own household chores. "The magnetic flux massages your muscles while you sleep. Before, I would wake up in the morning feeling like I had been slammed into concrete or hit by a car—my muscles were locked up stiff. Now they were unlocking, and it was wild. Magnets reduced my pain by sixty to seventy percent, and, unlike pain medication, they don't damage your liver or wear out." She ordered shoe pads that stopped her neuropathy—the burning sensation in her feet—and her foot pain. She wore Velcro magnet patches in her jeans pockets and put magnetic seat pads in her car.

Released from her private hell, Joy reveled in simply being able to function again, but was still always exhausted. She consulted Dr. Stephen Leighton, M.D., in Winston-Salem, North Carolina,[2] who had a reputation in four surrounding states for his success in treating fibromyalgia.

"I love this doctor. He takes you right back into his office and talks to you, and he really listens. He is a caring, wonderful person. I had never really gone to doctors before my illness, so I thought they knew all the answers. But now I realized, some of them graduated in the bottom of their class," she said and laughed, "and you don't know which one you're getting."

Dr. Leighton believed her problems were thyroid-related, so he ran the usual tests but gave equal attention to the symptoms she described. He told Joy about Wilson's thyroid syndrome, a condition in which thyroid tests may be in normal ranges but cells have become thyroid-resistant (described in greater detail below). He started Joy on specially compounded, slow-release T_3, the active form of thyroid hormone.

At home, Joy consulted her medical books and was amazed to find that lithium is known to cause pain throughout the body as a side effect and it is an antithyroid drug that blocks T_3 production. The first symptom of hypothyroidism is neuropathy, that burning, tingling, stinging in her feet, followed by muscle cramping that gets worse the longer antithyroid medicines are used.

Although doctors seemed not to know how lithium works, Joy quickly connected the dots. By blocking T_3 production, lithium lowers energy levels, slows metabolism, causing inevitable weight gain, and slows the brain, thus lowering mania. Even when the thyroid gland is shown to be producing adequate T_4 on test results, if the body can't convert the T_4 to T_3, then hypothyroidism results.

Joy found a new psychiatrist who agreed that lithium was interfering with her thyroid function and took her off the drug.

She continued Wilson's T_3 therapy with Dr. Leighton for several cycles and felt much better, but when she went off T_3 for two months to see if her own thyroid output would normalize, her body functions slowed again and symptoms returned. As they experimented, Dr. Leighton prescribed methadone to ease her discomfort. Used in the United States primarily to treat heroin addicts, low doses of methadone are commonly given in Europe for chronic pain. Joy preferred it to other painkillers since it wasn't addictive and didn't make her feel high, leaving her able to think clearly.

Joy started taking multivitamins and minerals, becoming aware of foods that inhibit thyroid function—soybean products, raw cruciferous vegetables (cabbage, cauliflower, broccoli), and unsaturated fats, such as safflower, corn, canola, and nut oils—and other antithyroid substances, such as excess estrogen, pesticides, fluoride, and mercury.

After several more T_3 cycles, where Joy's symptoms returned whenever she went off the compound, it became clear that her body could no longer make T_3, so Dr. Leighton put her on a permanent low dose. "Psychiatrists claim that once a patient is taken off lithium, the thyroid will come back to normal," says Joy, "but I don't think they know. I truly believe lithium damaged my thyroid. As long as I'm on the T_3, I continue to get better and have more energy."

I spoke with Joy again about a year after she had started the T_3. She was vibrant and excited as she said, "I went surfing the weekend before last! I surfed at Carolina Beach! Can you believe that? I had so much fun. I was told by all those doctors that I would have to learn to live in pain forever. I just wish they could have seen me."

Illnesses and Conditions That Foster Depression

AIDS, anemia, arthritis, Addison's disease, Asperger's syndrome, attention deficit hyperactivity disorder, brain tumors, bulimia, candida yeast infection, cancers (especially of the central nervous system), Cushing's disease, cerebrovascular disease, chronic pain, chronic fatigue syndrome, diabetes, epilepsy (temporal lobe), fibromyalgia, food allergies, heart disease, heavy metal toxicity, hepatitis, hyperthyroidism, hypoglycemia, hypothyroidism, influenza, Kleine-Levin syndrome, liver disease, lung disease, lupus, Lyme disease, menopause, mononucleosis, multiple sclerosis, pellagra, Parkinson's disease, porphyria, premenstrual syndrome, postviral flu syndrome, schizophrenia, sleep disturbances, stroke, syphilis, temporo-mandibular joint (TMJ) problems, tuberculosis, viral pneumonias, velo-cardio-facial syndrome, vitamin deficiencies, Wilson's disease.[3,4,5]

Categories or Classes of Drugs That Spawn Depression

Alpha-methyldopa, amphetamine (withdrawal), antibiotics, antidepressants, antihistamines, anti-inflammatory agents, antimalarials, antipsychotics (tranquilizers), arthritis medications, barbiturates, benzodiazepines, beta-blockers, birth control pills, chemotherapy medications, cholinergics, cimetidine, corticosteriods, cycloserine, diet pills, diuretics, estrogens and progesterone, heart medications, high blood pressure medications, indomethacin, levodopa, certain pain relievers, ranitidine, reserpine, sedatives, seizure medications, tranquilizers, vincristine.[6]

Safe Harbor's informative Web site, www.alternativementalhealth .com, gives a five-page list of depression-causing medications by generic and brand names.[7]

Ironically, many drugs that induce depression are those used to treat it. This makes sense when you realize that because these drugs affect specific neurotransmitters, and everyone's brain chemistry disorder is different, they help some individuals while making others' imbalances worse.

Diseases or Conditions That May Trigger Mania

AIDS	Mercury or metal toxicity
Brain tumors or head trauma	Neurosyphilis
Diabetes	Sodium imbalance
Epilepsy	Stress, severe
Hyperthyroidism	Systemic lupus
Hypothyroidism	Viral infections

Drugs That May Cause Manic Symptoms

Allergy medications

Antihistamines (high doses)

Cocaine or methamphetamines

Epinephrine in any medication

Quinolone (an antibiotic)

Steroids (high doses)

Why the Thyroid Is So Critical

Depression has long been linked with an underactive thyroid, a small gland in the neck just below the Adam's apple. The thyroid's vital function is regulation of both body temperature and metabolism through secretion of two major hormones: thyroxine (T_4) and triiodothyronine (T_3).

Most T_4 is converted to T_3 in the liver and kidneys. T_3 is the "active" form that works at the receptors in cells, affecting each cell's metabolic rate and, consequently, the entire body. Too little of these hormones (hypothyroidism) makes body processes run slow. Too much of these hormones (hyperthyroidism) pushes the body into overdrive, running too fast.

In addition to controlling temperature and metabolism, thyroid hormones impact energy production, weight, heart rate, cholesterol levels, and bone density. They affect sex drive, sleep, growth hormones, digestion, the immune system, and brain function. Persistent low thyroid contributes to diabetes, cancer, heart disease, gallbladder problems, fibromyalgia, and depression.[8,9]

Classic symptoms of low thyroid are depression, fatigue, and always feeling cold, especially in the hands and feet. Others symptoms are anxiety, mental sluggishness, slow or slurred speech, high or low blood pressure, weight gain or loss, slow wound healing, hypoglycemia, insomnia, migraines, increased allergic reactions, PMS and infertility, loss of sex drive, constipation, dry skin or acne, hoarseness, and hair loss, especially of outer eyebrows.

In the brain, the hypothalamus secretes TRH (thyrotropin-releasing hormone), which triggers the pituitary to release TSH (thyroid-stimulating hormone). Both TRH and TSH can be measured to check thyroid function. But many doctors believe blood levels may show normal ranges on tests even when there is a profound deficiency of thyroid hormone inside cells. Normal test results accompanied by obvious low thyroid symptoms is termed subclinical hypothyroidism.

A 1981 *Journal of the American Medical Association* study reported that 20 out of 250 consecutive patients referred for psychiatric evaluation had hypothyroidism and, of those 20, 50 percent showed *normal* TSH levels. A 2002 study of bipolar patients having a slow response to pharmaceutical treatments concluded, "Our results suggest that nearly three-quarters of patients with bipolar disorder have a thyroid profile that may be suboptimal for antidepressant response."[10] According to the August 3, 2002, issue of *The Lancet*, thyroid diagnostic problems may stem from using too broad laboratory ranges, which don't reflect the ideal level for a particular individual.[11]

Other doctors believe the problem is due to cellular thyroid resistance. An early study published in the *Annals of Internal Medicine* in 1977 showed that conversion of T_4 to T_3 decreases by as much as 50 percent during periods of fasting and severe illness. It is also more common in nationalities with a long ancestral history of famine: Scots, Irish, Welsh, Native American, and Russian.[12]

An enzyme converts T_4 to T_3 but becomes inhibited in response to famine or reduced calorie intake. As a result, inadequate conversion of T_4 to T_3 is almost universal in overweight people who have a history of dieting.[13] Any major stress, including trauma, surgery, or childbirth, can also be a cause. The conversion process may return to normal once the stress is relieved or it may be permanently altered.

Permanent changes in the conversion process may be caused by low body temperatures reducing enzyme activity. Metabolism—the internal chemical processes by which food is used for tissue growth or energy production—involves thousands of different enzymes, all of which are temperature-sensitive. When temperatures drop, all body processes slow down. Researchers have found decreased metabolic activity in the brain neurons of rats due to lowered body temperatures.[14]

In 1990, E. Denis Wilson, M.D., recognized the broad impact perpetually impaired conversion would have on health. Dubbing the condition Wilson's thyroid syndrome, he published a book by that title in 1991, outlining numerous ailments caused by this form of hypothyroidism and a way to correct it.[15] Although ignored or debunked by many doctors, cellular thyroid resistance was linked to mutations in the c-erbAβ gene on chromosome 3 in a study published in *Endocrine Reviews* in 1993.[16]

The easiest way to measure cellular resistance is to take your oral temperature immediately upon rising in the morning for two or three days (not during ovulation). Although 98.6°F is considered average normal oral temperature for adults, temperatures drop while you sleep, gradually rise in the morning, peak in the afternoon, and slowly drop again at night. A morning reading of 97.5–98.0°F or less, or low temperatures midday in the 96–97° range, may indicate a T_3 deficiency or cellular resistance.

Wilson's method of adjusting the body's thermostat, reestablishing normal T_4 to T_3 conversion, and relieving symptoms involves taking specially compounded, slow-release T_3[17] in capsules in a twenty-two-day cycle. The T_3 is then discontinued for at least two weeks between cycles. During the process, patients record temperature and pulse readings, marking the daily average on a graph.[18]

The goal is to establish a closer-to-normal temperature that the body will maintain even after medication is discontinued. Frequently, one cycle will raise the average temperature half a degree, or it may take three to five cycles to reach normal ranges. If the body's thermostat does not reset after several cycles and hypothyroid symptoms fail to subside, specially compounded T_3 supplementation or other thermoregulation strategies should be explored.

The body must have iodine to make thyroid hormones, which is why the U.S. government requires that table salt be iodized. Iodine is found in vegetables—if adequate amounts of iodine exist in the soil—and in kelp and other forms of seaweed, and in seafood. The amino acid tyrosine, found in protein, is also a precursor of thyroid hormones. At least one gram of tyrosine a day is necessary to prevent hypothyroidism and low adrenal function.[19] Certain vitamins and minerals are essential as well. Copper is required for the production of T_4; selenium and zinc are necessary for conversion to T_3; vitamins A, B-complex, C, and E, plus calcium, magnesium, manganese, and coenzyme Q10 are vital thyroid cofactors.

Additional Hormones That Impact Brain Function

Adrenal Hormones. Two crescent-shaped adrenal glands rest on top of the kidneys and produce over 150 different hormones responsible for maintaining critical bodily functions, such as salt and water balance, metabolism of carbohydrates, and regulation of blood sugar.[20] The adrenals manufacture adrenaline (also called epinephrine), a potent "fight or flight" hormone that causes blood to race to the brain, heart, and muscles, aiding survival in times of danger.

DHEA. A steroid released from the adrenal gland, DHEA (dehydroepiandrosterone) is the most abundant circulating hormone in humans, and influences over 150 known repair functions throughout the body and brain.[21] Touted by some as a powerful anti-aging factor, DHEA's actions are not completely understood, however, so controversy rages about whether or not to supplement low levels.

Deficiencies have been observed to result in low adaptability to stress, less energy, reduced sex drive, and compromised immunity. Scientists have found a strong correlation between low DHEA and hypothyroidism.[22] A 1986 study in the *New England Journal of Medicine* found that people with higher DHEA levels lived longer and had a much lower risk of heart disease.[23] Recent studies using DHEA supplements have also shown a reduction in abdominal fat, improved glucose metabolism, and increased insulin sensitivity.[24]

Insulin. Low blood glucose (sugar) resulting from release of too much insulin (a hormone produced by the pancreas) is called hypoglycemia and can cause dramatic mood fluctuations. It is usually related to eating too many carbohydrates with inadequate fiber supplies, or from excessive caffeine intake, but hypoglycemia can also result from low thyroid.[25] Low blood sugar symptoms include depression, irritability, anxiety, panic attacks, fatigue, headaches, trouble concentrating, insomnia, weakness, and tremors. When symptoms are relieved by food, it is a sure sign that hypoglycemia is involved.

Skipping breakfast, consuming too much caffeine, smoking, or eating mostly junk food all intensify blood sugar spikes, inevitably followed by low moods. Yet, hypoglycemics crave sweets and substances that give them a temporary energy high. Snacks every three hours containing high-fiber complex carbohydrates and small amounts of protein help maintain stable blood sugar levels and ease cravings. Supplements that enable people to go for longer periods between meals without a dip in blood sugar include daily chromium and the amino acid glutamine.[26]

Cortisol. Another adrenal hormone, cortisol is secreted in response to stress. In moderate amounts, it regulates immune response, counteracts insulin, and stimulates conversion of protein to the brain's fuel, glucose. Perpetual stress, however, generates too much cortisol, which leads to diminished conversion of thyroid T_4 into T_3.

According to Dharma Khalsa, M.D., author of *Brain Longevity*, constant stress is *toxic* to brain cells. Cortisol raises blood sugar temporarily, but too much inhibits its use by the brain's primary memory center, the hippocampus. Overabundant cortisol interferes with neurotransmitter function, impairing concentration and creating the temporary befuddlement that occurs under stress. Cortisol also disrupts brain cell metabolism by allowing too much calcium to enter cells, causing production of free radicals that kill from within.[27]

Constant stress and poor nutrition, endemic in our culture, weaken the adrenal glands. Frequently, people reach for a cup of coffee or a chocolate bar for a shot of energy, unaware that they are stimulating already exhausted glands. Adrenal insufficiency lowers immunity, disrupts blood sugar metabolism, causes fatigue, and interferes with normal sleep rhythms. When the adrenals are weak, thyroid medication will produce limited or transient improvement. Instead, work with trained holistic practitioners to repair adrenal function through a healthier balance of protein and carbohydrates, limiting sugars and avoiding allergens and stimulants like caffeine, diet pills, alcohol, and cigarettes.

Melatonin. Sunlight impacts the pineal, a light-sensitive gland in the brain that connects to the body's circadian rhythm, our "biological clock." Absence of light stimulates production of the hormone melatonin, with levels peaking around midnight and falling toward dawn, influencing whether we feel sleepy or awake.

In an intriguing book titled *Sync*, author Steve Strogatz, a researcher who has served on the faculties of Harvard, MIT, and Cornell, says the body's biological clock marches in lockstep with body temperature cycles, and that body temperature determines when we fall asleep, the duration of sleep, and our level of alertness (which again reinforces the importance of thyroid and temperature regulation). Later studies have demonstrated that short-term memory, secretion of melatonin, and several other cognitive and physiological functions have synergistic relationships with the temperature cycle and to one another.

According to Strogatz, research in the 1970s pinpointed two clusters of neurons in the front of the brain's hypothalamus as the master clock control. Recent work points to molecular circadian rhythms with interlocking biochemical feedback loops that involve DNA transcription and eight clock genes. How electrical activity is synchronized throughout the body, however, is still unknown, although "chemical diffusion of a neurotransmitter called GABA" is suspected.[28]

Melatonin is believed to synchronize the secretion of other hormones. It decreases the stress hormone cortisol, stimulates brain-calming GABA, enhances production of thyroid hormones, promotes deep sleep, protects DNA, reduces blood coagulation, increases natural killer cells, and promotes zinc utilization. It even is said to slow hair graying.[29]

Tryptophan from protein becomes serotonin, a precursor to melatonin production. Levels are suppressed, however, by caffeine, tobacco, alcohol, chocolate, aspirin, SSRI antidepressants, tranquilizers, sleep medications, or taking B-complex too close to bedtime.[30] Resulting disrupted sleep cycles, if prolonged, can easily trigger psychiatric symptoms.

Seasonal affective disorder (SAD) is a type of depression brought on by too much melatonin in response to longer hours of darkness in northern climates. SAD is found in only 1.5 percent of Florida residents but in roughly 10 percent of New Hampshire residents.[31] With this disorder, people crave carbohydrates, gain weight, sleep more, lose interest in sex, become withdrawn, and generally act as though they were in a mild state of hibernation. For some sufferers, full-spectrum lights, on a timer, that simulate an early dawn or extended dusk fool the body. For me, taking omega-3 fish oils quickly ended both clinical depression and SAD.

Estrogen. Estrogen causes calories to be transformed into fat; thyroid hormone turns fat into energy. When women eat more calories than needed or have excess fat, estrogen production escalates. Diets in wealthy countries, high in fats, sugar, refined starches, and processed foods, lead to estrogen levels in women twice those found in women living in developing nations.

In the brain, estrogen promotes mood-regulating neurotransmitters, particularly serotonin, making it both an antidepressant and a sleep promoter. Too much estrogen, however (especially when not balanced by adequate progesterone), interferes with thyroid function and can lead to depression. Excessive estrogen levels also increase blood clotting, impair blood sugar stability, cause loss of zinc and retention of copper (an imbalance contributing to mania, violence, and obsessive disorders), and reduce oxygen levels in all cells, elevating the risk of cancer and autoimmune disorders.[32]

Birth control pills are one source of excess estrogen that may throw other hormones out of balance. Contents vary by brand, but oral contraceptives contain patented synthetic estrogen substitutes (totally different from the body's natural estrogen), along with a similarly altered progesterone substitute called progestin. These suppress ovulation along with thyroid, human growth, and testosterone hormones.[33]

Birth control pills deplete the body of vitamin B_6 and elevate copper, which may trigger mania, paranoia, or hallucinations. The pills deplete magnesium, which is necessary for release and uptake of serotonin, increasing anxiety, depression, or insomnia. Anyone on birth control pills should take extra B-vitamins along with supplemental magnesium and zinc, to keep copper in balance.[34]

Xenoestrogens are foreign substances originating outside the body that have hormonelike and estrogenlike activity in the body. Nearly all are derived from petroleum. They are fat-soluble, nonbiodegradable, and accumulate in fatty tissues—the breast, brain, and liver. They are ubiquitous in pesticides, sprayed on lawns or gardens, and in the food chain are sprayed on fruits, produce, and corn fed to animals that end up as the meat we eat. Xenoestrogens are in detergents, dishwashing liquids, hair and skin care products, medicines, perfume, and plastics, some of which shed these substances when heated. Avoid using plastics in the microwave or water bottles left in the sun.[35]

Estrogen dominance, where progesterone is low, whether from physical, food, medical, or environmental sources, mimics low thyroid, increasing the risk of depression, allergies, weight gain, and cancer.[36] As a result, unnatural intake of estrogen should be avoided, especially synthetic versions in hormone replacement therapy or pesticides. Estrogen should always be balanced by *natural* progesterone.

Progesterone. This is an essential hormone made from cholesterol. Yes, that much-maligned substance we have been told to avoid in our diet. In fact, all hormones are made from cholesterol. The body's production line goes like this: Cholesterol is used to make pregnenolone, which is converted to DHEA and progesterone. From these the body makes various estrogens, testosterone, and steroid hormones.[37] Low-cholesterol diets that were supposed to protect our hearts (which some new research refutes) can cause low levels of *all* hormones, our body regulators. Even given adequate cholesterol, hormone production drops dramatically as we age. There is roughly a 50 percent diminishment by age fifty and an almost 100 percent decline by age seventy-five.[38]

Postpartum depression, which affects an estimated 13 percent of new mothers,[39] may be related to adrenal exhaustion following childbirth, but it is most often linked to an extreme drop in progesterone. Research in Wales found that, among 120 women, those with the highest prebirth and the lowest postbirth progesterone levels had the worst postpartum depression.

According to Uzzi Reiss, M.D., O.B./Gyn., author of *Natural Hormone Balance for Women* and a man who has delivered thousands of babies, "towering hormonal levels during pregnancy come crashing down after childbirth," with progesterone falling to nearly zero. For a new mother suffering from depression, even suicidal thoughts, he strongly recommends one 200-milligram injection of natural progesterone each day during her hospital stay or until her moods return to normal, which usually occurs within eight to twelve hours after an injection. With the progesterone injections he prescribes a 0.1-milligram natural estrogen patch, because estrogen levels also drop drastically after childbirth. When the patient returns home, he switches her to a basic natural estrogen formula he has used for years, called Tri-Estrogen.[40]

Natural progesterone is an antidepressant. It facilitates thyroid function, helps to build bone, normalizes blood sugar levels, and restores sex drive as well as helping to use fat for energy. It restores proper cell oxygen levels, protecting against fibrocystic breasts, and helps prevent endometrial and breast cancer.

Testosterone. A precursor to the estrogens, testosterone promotes stamina, strong muscles, less body fat, sturdy bones, and feelings of security and stability. Excess testosterone results in aggressive behavior, oily skin, acne, loss of head hair, and growth of facial hair.[41]

Balancing Hormones

Depression, mania, poor memory, and confusion can all result from deficiencies or excesses of hormones. As indicated by this brief discussion, their actions and interactions are so complex that scientists and doctors still have great gaps in their understanding. Since hormones regulate vital body functions, do not take synthetic (that is, patented) hormones because they are incompatible with your body, and never supplement with any natural substance without first having your hormone levels tested. Natural hormone supplements are available over the counter, but this is not an area to do-it-yourself.

Find a naturopathic doctor who has a great deal of experience using natural hormone therapy or a conventionally trained physician who has rejected synthetic pharmaceutical versions and become an expert in natural options. Request thyroid blood tests (TSH, T_3, T_4, TRH, and antithyroglobulin and antithyroperoxidase), and if they are all normal but your symptoms are not, take your temperature and read about Wilson's thyroid syndrome. To determine other hormone levels, many holistic doctors consider saliva testing the most accurate, since only the free, or active, forms of hormones get into saliva.

CHAPTER 4

Rebuilding with Glyconutrients, Proteins, and Amino Acids

"The norm in life was for me to come home from school and find my mom in bed at 3:30 in the afternoon, all the windows covered, lights off, with a pillow over her head," says Haley Hartford. "I had no concept that depression wasn't a part of everyday life."

That changed, however, when Haley left for college. "I began to see the world differently—that my life had not been 'normal.' I struggled with mild depression that continued all through college, but I fought and ignored the signs because I was *not* going to become my mother. I was determined to be 'normal.'"

A few years after college, following a brief courtship, Haley got married. It only took a few weeks for her to realize that life was not going to be the fairy tale she had imagined. There were a great number of unforeseen problems. "My husband was unemployed and having difficulty finding a job," she says with a laugh that still betrays a hint of the bitterness she felt. "I got more and more depressed, but I thought my depression was completely situational. It eventually got to the point where I was just unable to control the way I was feeling."

A doctor prescribed Zoloft. "I was really terrified. I came home from the doctor that day and threw my prescription at my husband, who was occupying his usual place on the couch, as if to say, 'Do you see what you've driven me to?' I was so angry . . . and so scared. I was afraid that the Zoloft would make me a zombie, but it really seemed to help. It evened me out so that I didn't have the huge ups and downs, but I also didn't have any of the emotions I used to. I'm a very emotional person, and I lost some piece of that."

Worse still, over time Haley became self-destructive in spite of the antidepressant, not an unusual occurrence for psychiatric patients. When I asked her to explain, if she could, what drove her to hurt herself, there was a long pause and a deep breath before she spoke.

"That's one of those things that's still a little difficult for me to talk about. I didn't take a razor blade or anything like that. I would bite myself, leaving huge bruises on my arms. When I would go into a tailspin where I felt like my world was falling apart, I would find a place on my arm and bite. Another thing I would do was break candles or glasses, pick up the shards, and just squeeze them in my hands until I would cut my hands. I remember one particularly nasty altercation with my husband: I was beating my own head against the wall, trying to knock myself out because the pain of what I was feeling was so intense that I just wanted to go to sleep to escape.

"The [emotional] pain of what I was going through was so bad, the only way I could deal with it was to concentrate it into something physical. This one physical pain on one specific part of my body was all of a sudden manageable."

Zoloft also reduced her sex drive, which as a newlywed with an already rocky marriage was not good.

Within a year, however, Haley's husband found a job and the relationship got better. She thought the situational depression was over, so she could get off the medicine. After consulting with her doctor, she tried the step-down withdrawal process, but "Every time I came off of it, the depression came roaring back with a vengeance. I was in tailspin after tailspin. It got to the point where my doctor gave me Xanax because coming off the depression drug made my anxiety so bad I was even more self-destructive. I could see it was this incredible cycle that would have no end.

"I tried probably six times to come off depression meds, but each time I would have some horrible episode. I was never suicidal, but when the episode passed and I was a little more clearheaded, the fear struck me: 'What if next time, I take it one step too far?'"

Haley, a striking redhead with blue eyes, fair skin, and freckles, once outgoing and vivacious, cut off all contact with friends or anyone who might notice how much she had changed. In her mind, at age twenty-six, she had become her mother.

Except her mother had experienced a remarkable improvement as a result of working with Neecie Moore, Ph.D., a therapist in Carrollton, Texas. Dr. Neecie has spent twenty years helping people remove "roadblocks" to better living and authoring nine books, including *What's a Nice Person Like Me Doing in a Body Like This.*[1]

Observing her mother's progress, Haley consulted Dr. Neecie too. In addition to therapy, Haley was introduced to glyconutrients (special sugars, discussed below) in "Dr. Neecie's Depression Cocktail," a blend of these sugars with other natural nutrients. According to the doctor, the depression cocktail has been 85 percent successful in getting depressed, bipolar, and other patients off psychiatric medications entirely.

Haley started taking the depression cocktail in July, but admits that she was not diligent about following the regimen. Then in early December, her husband announced that he wanted a divorce. Haley's world collapsed, but her personal transformation began. "I decided that, above all else, no matter what, I had lost my marriage, I had lost my husband, but my emotional health was going to become my first priority. I'm getting out of this cycle, whatever it takes."

She went back to taking the nutrient cocktail on January 2, 2005, and on January 5 stopped taking all depression and anxiety medications. "I was still emotional—with the separation happening right before Christmas and New Year's, and with a complicated divorce that took several months, but what I noticed was that the emotions were manageable. It's hard to explain, but I can *feel* when my hormones are swinging all over the place—it's almost a physical sensation—and I didn't feel that anymore. I calmed [down] and things just evened out to where I felt like I was taking control for the first time.

"Every other time I had tried to come off my meds, I had these horrible side effects of dizziness, nausea, and vertigo, like I was on a Tilt-a-Whirl. When I started the glyconutrients and stopped the meds cold turkey, I never had a side effect once."

Dr. Neecie's nutrient cocktail consisted of Mannatech[2] products: Ambrotose™, a blend of eight essential sugars; Sport, a wild Mexican yam source of DHEA; AmbroStart®, an energizing, orange-flavored powder that is mixed with water to create a fruity beverage; and Mannatonin™, a blend of ingredients that support the body's natural melatonin production, aiding repairs that occur only in deep sleep. To these, Haley added a vitamin and mineral supplement, GlycoLEAN® Catalyst containing Ambroglycin® (an amino acid bonded with Ambrotose™ complex to the minerals), designed to support the body's ability to use fat.

The nutrients healed more than just her depression and anxiety. "I dropped thirty pounds because of the glyconutrients," she says. Always a sickly person, "I made it through a winter without bronchitis for the first time since I was five years old. Instead of worrying about whatever my current sickness was, I wasn't fighting symptoms anymore. It was, 'I feel okay. Wow, it's so new!'"

Haley now works as a certified life coach, teaching the power of scripture-based counseling. "I wish I could tell you my life's been perfect since. It hasn't. But it's been manageable. I've been able to maintain a level of control of my emotions. I feel like I'm taking responsibility for my life instead of depending on some drug that's going to zombie me out so I don't *feel* anything. I'm focused. I'm motivated. I've been able to find meaning in helping other people deal with what I'm dealing with. It gives me a lot of credibility when I can say, 'You know what, I was there.'"

The Body's Building Materials

Neurotransmitters are made from proteins, which are chains of amino acids whose arrangement determines whether the protein is used as an enzyme, a hormone, an oxygen carrier, or for muscular contraction or cell regeneration. Amino acids are considered the building blocks of the body, while enzymes are the catalysts that trigger virtually all biochemical processes. Both are derived from protein. Until roughly twenty years ago, scientists also believed proteins were the primary communication molecules. Now they think differently, based on studies of glyconutrients, or vital sugars.

The first international conference on this cutting-edge field of science known as glycobiology was held in 1989 at the University of California, Los Angeles. Nobel Prizes were awarded in 1991, 1994, and 1999 for work related to this cellular communication process. In 1996, the American Naturopathic Medical Association recognized Bill II. McAnalley, Ph.D., and H. Reginald McDaniel, Ph.D. (co-inventors of the glyconutrient base for Mannatech's supplements, used by Haley) with the "Discovery of the Year Award" for their work on glyconutrients.[3]

Science Magazine's March 23, 2001, issue dedicated twelve articles to educating the science and medical community about glyconutrients, glycobiology, and glycoscience. The Massachusetts Institute of Technology published a feature in its *Technology Review* on the "Ten Emerging Technologies That Will Change the World," including how these sugars determine the function of proteins.

What are glyconutrients? Out of two hundred known saccharides (sugars), there are eight single sugar molecules (monosaccharides) that are necessary for health. The eight, collectively called glyconutrients, attach and form "fingers" on the ends of protein molecules. Every cell requires glycoproteins for 85 percent of its cellular processes.[4] Glycoproteins are the building blocks of the immune system, where cellular communication determines which entities in the body are tagged as friend or foe.[5]

Cells talk, it seems, in intricate sugar codes. When two cells touch, these tiny sugar molecules confer with their neighbors.[6] Because of this interaction on the cell's surface, hormones do not have to enter cells to turn on various functions, which explains why minute quantities are sufficient.[7]

Glycoproteins are so vital for normal development of the human nervous system that human breast milk contains five of the eight sugars, or glyconutrients, in significant quantities, giving an infant protection against infections and nourishment that no other formula or mammal's milk can offer.[8]

Insufficient intake of essential sugars in adults is slowly being recognized as the fundamental cellular problem underlying vastly different ailments. A deficiency can cause either too great an immune response, as in allergic conditions or autoimmune diseases, or too little immune reaction, so natural killer cells fail to recognize diseased or cancerous cells and destroy them.

Two of the eight monosaccharides, glucose and galactose, are available in most diets:

Glucose is the most common single sugar molecule and the primary brain fuel. Table sugar, a two-sugar molecule (or disaccharide) composed of fructose and glucose, lacks the nutrients necessary for its own use, making fruits and starchy vegetables better glucose sources. The ability to metabolize glucose is altered in some cases of depression and eating disorders. Adult-onset diabetics also have difficulty absorbing glucose because perpetual overabundance has made cells resistant to it.[9]

Galactose is converted by the body from lactose, the natural sugar in milk and dairy products. Figs, grapes, black-eyed peas, tomatoes, hazelnuts, and many kinds of beans are also rich in galactose.[10] Needed for proper immune function (especially in arthritis and lupus), galactose inhibits tumor growth, aids wound healing, retards cataracts, and maintains healthy colonic bacteria.

Galactolipids (galactose plus fat) are found on myelin sheaths that insulate nerve fibers. Glycoproteins on nerve cells are receptors of the neurotransmitters, including norepinephrine, dopamine, and serotonin. Disrupted reception can cause mood disorders or abnormal movements, as in Parkinson's disease.

In theory, the body can manufacture any of the six less available sugars from glucose or galactose, assuming, of course, that you have the enzymes needed and your metabolic pathways are working right. But enzyme conversions require high levels of energy and can be interrupted by toxins, stress, drugs, processed foods, lack of specific enzymes, and age. Glyconutrient supplementation frees up enzyme supplies to do other vital conversions.

The six glyconutrients not so likely to be a part of our diet contribute to our health in intriguing ways.

Fucose is found in several medicinal mushrooms, some seaweeds like kelp and wakame, and beer yeast. It is important in brain development, neurotransmission, and may improve the ability to create long-term memories. Active against herpes viruses, it guards against respiratory infections and inhibits allergic reactions, inflammation, and cancer growth, as well as aiding collagen production.[11] According to the work of Doris Lefkowitz, Ph.D., severe rheumatoid arthritis has been linked to low galactose and fucose levels.[12] Fucose metabolism is abnormal in cystic fibrosis, diabetes, and cancer.[13]

N-acetylgalactosamine, the least studied, is found in bovine and shark cartilage and red algae. Absorbed from the intestine, it is particularly concentrated in the brain and nerve tissue and has antiviral, antitumor actions.[14]

Xylose is found in guava, pears, berries, aloe vera, kelp, echinacea, psyllium, broccoli, spinach, eggplant, peas, green beans, oleva, cabbage, and corn. It serves as a cell membrane receptor, has antibacterial and antifungal properties, and is especially helpful against candida (see chapter 6), promoting growth of friendly bacteria in the intestines.[15]

Mannose is found in aloe vera leaf gel, fenugreek seed, carob gum, guar gum, black or red currants, gooseberries, green beans, cayenne pepper, shitake mushrooms, kelp, cabbage, eggplant, tomatoes, and turnips. It is the foundation of all the vital sugars, needed for many fundamental cell activities. Mannose modulates the immune system, is an anti-inflammatory that eases rheumatoid arthritis and lupus, lowers blood sugar and triglyceride levels in diabetics, acts to prevent some types of bacterial infections, suppresses tumor growth, and may inhibit tumor cell metastasis.[16, 17]

N-acetylglucosamine (NAG) is best known as glucosamine, its derivative, a building block of cartilage. NAG is available in bovine and shark cartilage, shitake mushrooms, and shells of crustaceans like shrimp and crab. Most of the studies of NAG have been conducted with glucosamine, known to repair cartilage while reducing osteoarthritis. It also decreases insulin secretion, is an immune modulator with antitumor and antiviral properties (active against HIV),[18] and is believed to play a role in transport of the iodine-containing glycoprotein used in thyroid function.[19]

N-acetylneuraminic acid (NANA) is found in whey protein and chicken eggs. Especially important for brain development and learning, it has been shown in animal studies to improve both memory and performance. Involved in the metabolism of fats, NANA affects the thickness of mucus that serves as a defense against bacteria, viruses, and other pathogens. A 1995 issue of *Antimicrobial Agents and Chemotherapy* reported that an N-acetylneuraminic acid mixture was up to a thousand times more effective in fighting the influenza virus than antiviral drugs.[20] NANA also influences blood thickening and cholesterol levels, lowering LDL—the bad one.[21]

Many tree and plant substances contain multiple glyconutrients: aloe vera, aribinogalactan from the larch tree, astragalus, gum acacia, gum ghatti, limu moui, medicinal mushrooms, and fruit pectins.[22]

Although clinical studies of glyconutrients and depression in humans have yet to be conducted, it is known that glucose levels in people with chronic depression, anorexia or bulimia, obsessive-compulsive disorder, and schizophrenia are often lower than those in people without these disorders. In bipolar disorder, both high and low glucose levels have been found.[23]

One small, six-month study of glyconutritional supplementation in twenty children with bipolar disorder showed that almost all the children had a reduction in the severity of their bipolar symptoms and several experienced improved ability to tolerate psychotropic medications and reduced adverse effects from the medications.[24]

Mannatech, the manufacturer of all the supplements Haley used, was founded in 1994 and is the leading producer of glyconutrients today. Its chief science officer, Dr. Bill McAnnalley, was one of the first to recognize the benefits of nutritional supplements containing a blend of saccharides that would enhance intercellular communications. Thanks to Dr. McAnnalley's extensive career in pharmacology, the company chose not to develop synthetic carbohydrates but instead to focus research and development on all-natural saccharide supplements, which are fully compatible with the body's innate systems. Mannatech patented the supplements' composition and use instead of creating an altered molecule, like drugs. It was a brilliant move that has taken the now publicly traded company global in just ten years and made it an envied leader in the emerging wellness industry.

Essential Amino Acids

Eight amino acids are "essential," required by the body to function, but they cannot be produced internally. These amino acids are totally derived from diet: histidine, isoleucine, leucine, lysine, methionine, phenylalanine, tryptophan, and valine.[25] In theory, nonessential amino acids can be produced by the body from the essential ones. But some, such as tyrosine and cysteine, may not be synthesized in sufficient quantities for optimum brain function by people who have genetic metabolism flaws.

Malabsorption of nutrients is very common among the mentally ill, making adequate protein consumption crucial. Yet too much protein can contribute to osteoporosis. Protein consumed in amounts higher than those used by the body each day is not stored like fat, but rather is dumped into the urine, making it acidic. To buffer this acidity, the kidneys add calcium. If not enough calcium is in the diet each day, calcium stored in bones is withdrawn. While advertising gives the impression that osteoporosis is caused solely by insufficient calcium, a diet with an imbalance of protein or too much refined sugar, caffeine, and phosphorus from soft drinks can also be a culprit.[26]

Animal sources of protein, such as meat, poultry, fish, or dairy products, contain roughly 25 to 30 percent protein; beans, peas, and nuts are 10 to 12 percent protein; and vegetables range from 3 to 10 percent protein. Four to eight ounces of animal protein daily usually delivers what is needed (although athletes and people recovering from illness or surgery need more).[27] But do not fill your plate with potatoes, bread, pasta, white rice, and processed carbohydrates either, since these lead to obesity, diabetes, and heart disease. Vegetables are carbohydrates too—the really important ones. To feed your brain, eat mounds of vegetables and leafy greens, moderate amounts of legumes (peas, beans) and animal protein, small servings of *whole* grains, and fruits in place of desserts.

A few amino acids are especially vital to mental health. All are available by eating protein, but, as you will see from subsequent chapters, metabolism errors or faulty digestion often make supplements a good idea.

Tryptophan. Used to produce the calming neurotransmitter serotonin, along with adrenaline, dopamine, and GABA, tryptophan aids concentration and helps relieve depression, mania, stress, anxiety, irritability, and insomnia. Vitamin B_6 is necessary for the formation of tryptophan, and in turn, serotonin.[28]

For thirty years, tryptophan supplements were a safe, effective treatment for insomnia, but showed mixed success when used for depression. In 1989, one batch from a Japanese manufacturer became contaminated, causing thirty-six deaths. Although the problem was quickly solved, consumers must now get prescription tryptophan (paying more, of course) or use 5-HTP (5-hydroxytryptophan), a form extracted from an African plant seed.

The good news is that 5-HTP is a more reliable natural treatment for depression than tryptophan supplements. The body makes tryptophan into 5-HTP and then turns 5-HTP into serotonin. While only 3 percent of an oral dose of tryptophan is converted into serotonin, over 70 percent of 5-HTP is converted. Numerous double-blind studies have proved 5-HTP to be as effective as SSRI drugs like Prozac, Paxil, and Zoloft, while it is less expensive, better tolerated, and with fewer side effects.[29] Five-HTP also improves the quality of sleep, while antidepressants disrupt sleep patterns.

Methionine. This amino acid assists in the breakdown of fats and helps lower blood levels of histamine that, when elevated, contribute to mania, anxiety, and schizophrenia. It contains sulfur, which aids in detoxification, and it is a powerful antioxidant that inactivates free radicals.

Normally, methionine is used by the brain to manufacture all the SAMe (S-adenoxyl-methionine) it needs for methylation, the intricate biochemical process discussed in chapter 1. In some people, however, SAMe synthesis is impaired, reducing levels of serotonin and dopamine, and impairing the process that binds neurotransmitters to receptor sites, contributing to mental disorders.[30]

Cysteine and Cystine. These molecules are closely related and capable of converting into each other, as needed. Made from methionine, both contain sulfur, which promotes healthy skin and detoxification. Effective antioxidants and membrane stabilizers,[31] these amino acids are precursors to glutathione, which protects the liver and brain from toxic damage. Vitamin B_6 is essential for synthesis of these molecules.[32]

Phenylalanine. This amino acid is first converted into tyrosine, which is then used by the body to make dopamine and norepinephrine—neurotransmitters promoting alertness, elevating mood, aiding memory, decreasing pain, and suppressing the appetite.[33] Phenylalanine is also converted to phenylethylamine (PEA), a stimulant and antidepressant present in chocolate too (which is why we crave it so). Low urinary PEA levels are found in depressed patients, while elevated levels are found in schizophrenic patients.[34] L-phenylalanine is the supplement form recommended for stabilizing moods. The D-L-phenylalanine form relieves both chronic pain and depression.[35]

Tyrosine. A precursor to the stimulating neurotransmitters dopamine and norepinephrine, tyrosine is made from phenylalanine and combats depression. It increases PEA levels and aids in stress management. Just as important, tyrosine attaches to iodine atoms to form vital thyroid hormones. Low tyrosine levels are associated with hypothyroidism. If supplements are used, this amino acid should be taken with a high-carbohydrate meal or on an empty stomach, since it competes with tryptophan to cross the blood-brain barrier.[36]

Glutamine and Glutamate. Glutamine and glutamate are both forms of the nonessential amino acid glutamic acid.[37] Glutamine is the most common amino acid in the human body and is significant brain fuel, easily passing through the blood-brain barrier. But only small amounts of glutamine are found in foods. Glutamic acid, by contrast, is abundant, particularly in plant foods, so the body compensates by converting glutamic acid into glutamine, as needed. Glutamine promotes intelligence and memory, as well as the maintenance of a healthy digestive tract, decreasing intestinal permeability (leaky gut [see chapter 5]). It reduces alcohol and sugar cravings, moderates hypoglycemia, builds muscle, aids in fat metabolism, and supports mineral absorption, all while reducing depression, fatigue, and pain.[38,39]

Glutamic Acid. Three nonessential amino acids—glutamic acid, cysteine, and glycine—are linked to form glutathione peroxidase, the most important and abundant antioxidant enzyme the body makes. Antioxidants play defense in the body's fight against destructive free radicals, which are produced during the detoxification of harmful substances (more on this in chapter 6).[40] Toxins from outside the body, such as mercury, lead, or pesticides, are obviously dangerous, but the body produces its own toxins too—internally generated trash, such as hormones no longer needed, used neurotransmitters, or molecules tagged for elimination by a vigilant immune system. Glutamic acid provides the only means the brain has of detoxifying ammonia, a natural by-product of protein metabolism. This amino acid is also used for the metabolism of sugars and fats, and is a precursor of the calming neurotransmitter GABA (gamma-aminobutyric acid).

Taurine. A building block of all other amino acids, taurine is also a key component of bile, the substance needed for fat digestion and absorption of fat-soluble vitamins. Found in concentrations up to four times greater in children's brains than those of adults, taurine has a protective effect, and as a supplement is used to treat anxiety, epilepsy, hyperactivity, Down's syndrome, and seizures. Zinc deficiency and alcoholism can cause excessive loss of taurine through excretion in the urine, and diabetes increases the body's requirements for it. Not found in vegetable proteins, taurine can be made from cysteine or methionine as long as vitamin B_6 is present. So vegetarians or people with genetic metabolic disorders should take supplements.

Certain amino acids should not be supplemented if you have high blood pressure, Graves' disease, melanoma, migraines, ulcers, severe liver or kidney problems, or are pregnant, nursing, or taking certain medications. Always consult your doctor before using these natural supplements and discontinue them immediately if you experience any discomfort.[41]

Amino acids are readily available in all protein foods, with animal sources having the most concentrated levels, followed by beans, nuts and seeds, and then vegetables. *Nutrition Almanac* contains seventy fascinating pages of charts detailing the vitamins, minerals, and essential amino acids present in both natural and prepared foods.[42]

CHAPTER 5

Hidden Triggers: Allergies, Food Sensitivities, and Flawed Digestion

At the Safe Harbor Non-Pharma alternative mental health practitioners conference, Mary Jensen stood out because of her insightful questioning of each speaker and because she is also six-foot-four. Her personal story of recovery from depression is gripping.

When Mary moved to New York in 1973 to begin nurse's training, most of the patients she worked with were terminally ill, often comatose. One day as she walked into the room of a woman, a former schoolteacher, it was filled with spirits of children. "They were sitting on the radiator, sitting on the bed, perched on the head of the bed, on the pillows, and on the floor." Mary thought this meant she had a "spiritual gift," and although a practicing Catholic, she didn't find the phenomenon particularly distressing. "I just thanked them for being present and said I'd do my best with the patient."

By the next year, seeing spirits had become a common occurrence. Regular otherworldly occupants of her apartment were a woman and a dog. "It was all rather distracting," Mary said. "I would be trying to study when suddenly they would walk through the wall. I decided to call the woman Elizabeth. I'd come home after work and call out to my husband, 'Honey, I'm home,' then say, 'Oh, hi, Elizabeth. How's the dog?'"

Mary also began experiencing more frequent periods of emotional ups and downs, and she developed asthma. "It never occurred to me that I had an illness or that I should do something to make the spirits go away." Looking back years later, she believes this "second sight" was triggered by the loss of her only child in 1973, stress, and unknown environmental toxins. "I asked my mother if I was a child who had imaginary friends, but I'm one of twelve kids and she couldn't remember exactly who saw what," Mary says, and laughs.

Although Mary continued to work as a nurse and go to graduate school, such experiences remained part of her everyday life during ten years in New York. "I would hear my name called and feel like something was on my skin or rubbing the tips of my hair. In bed at night, I would see colored lights, little gyroscopes floating in the air in clusters, darting back and forth and up and down. I was always aware of lots of thoughts that after a while became a stream of noise with a flavor of negative criticism, disdain, and distress." Upon completing her master's degree, she accepted a job in Chicago as the nursing manager, overseeing a staff of fifty in a large geriatric rehabilitation facility. After she moved, the visions and sensations stopped completely, as did the asthma, but the depression and internal stream of negativity continued.

In the 1970s, the women's liberation movement was preaching that women should accept challenging jobs and live apart from their husbands, if necessary, so they would not be defined by or held back by marriage. "I got caught up in that nonsense and moved to Chicago, leaving my husband in New York, unaware that my life was out of control," says Mary. With a thousand miles between them, Mary was unable to see that her husband was ill, and the couple soon divorced. When he died suddenly from complications of alcoholism, Mary says, "I spent a lot of time crying and was inconsolable."

Very pious as a child, Mary had memorized the Latin mass in three or four versions and learned how to sew in order to make vestments to practice the mass at home. As a child, she would often faint as a result of the fasting required in those days and fall to the floor, hitting anything in the way. Now, in her thirties, she continued to seek comfort in her religion, but all she could do in church was cry. "There is part of a service where the words translated are 'through my fault, through my fault, through my own grievous fault,' and I would just dissolve into tears after that." Church became a symbol of something frightening and a reminder of what a terrible person she was, a feeling that persisted no matter what denomination or service she attended.

Mary attributed deepening depression to multiple stresses. "I think the underlying issue was that for over forty years I felt 'hopeless.' I always had a sense of doom—that there was something terribly wrong with me and if I found out what, I wouldn't be able to live through it."

It's easy to see how a girl who grew quickly to a full height of six-foot-four might feel like a misfit. Always stared at, often laughed at, she was expected to be an athlete or model but she wasn't very good at either. With a nearly photographic memory, however, Mary did well in school. "I immersed myself in learning. Since I was going to stand out, I was determined to have some sense of mastery." Yet, she did so quietly. "I expected to be ridiculed, for what I thought as well as for my size, so I didn't talk much."

At age thirty-five, she met Allen, on a blind date arranged by a mutual friend. Her job (now as a psychiatric nurse) was still very stressful, and he was a practitioner of Mahikari no Waza, the ancient art of spiritual purification by divine light energy known as Sukuinushi-sama.[1] Allen would call for a date, to see a movie or go out to dinner, and stop by to pick up Mary. Since she was usually exhausted or stressed out, he offered to "give her light" by chanting a prayer to God for spiritual purification, then raising his palm twelve inches from specific areas of the body for a few minutes each. Totally relaxed as a result of the process, she would fall asleep. "I was a real hot date," she says and chuckles.

Allen would close the door, go home, and call her the next day to arrange another get-together. "After this went on for about a month, he said, 'Look, I'm not going to give you light anymore. I want a date!' He took me to the local spiritual center where I could receive light any time."

Receiving spiritual purification by Mahikari no Waza calmed Mary. After several months of this spiritual practice, Mary decided to learn the art as well. She became surprised when, within a year, it had some "unintentional side effects." For one, she realized her inability to feel any sensations in the lower right quadrant of her back had been healed and all feeling restored. Her sense of feeling cold year-round improved too. Yet, her bouts of hopelessness persisted.

She and Allen married. His health declined soon afterward. He managed to continue working, but could do little else. The situation deteriorated further when his mother had a stroke and both his parents moved in with the couple. Mary gave up her career, becoming a full-time caregiver. She describes that year simply as "very difficult."

"My feelings of hopelessness got worse and worse. I just didn't feel there was any way out. I had deep, dark thoughts and wished my husband were dead." Oddly, she never became suicidal herself. "I always figured there was a reason why I was attracted to people who had huge challenges in their life that were not apparent until after I married them. I just believed that all things are for the good no matter what."

The director of the Sukyo Mahikari Center suggested that Mary spend time working on her own spiritual development by coming to give light at the center. "Little by little, I was able to develop gratitude for the seriousness of the condition I was in, rather than disdain for the mess I was in," she recalls. "With the developing of gratitude, I tried to tune in to what God wanted me to do. It became very basic. How do I be a wife to my husband without wishing he were dead?" His parents stayed only a year, but Allen's condition continued for twelve long years. Yet, through her spiritual practice, Mary was "able to become much more happy, even though nothing had changed."

In 1999, after Allen intensified his spiritual training, his decline reversed completely. It was as if a door had opened. He began exploring things like poor diet, water quality, and environmental factors that might be contributing to the couple's illnesses. Together they started on a path to wellness.

Over the next several years they gave light as much as possible, stopped smoking, eliminated from their diet all sugar, all forms of monosodium glutamate (MSG), caffeine, artificial sweeteners, milk products, and they cut down on wheat. They stopped drinking tap water, got rid of all known sources of fluoride, and started eating "as whole and natural as possible," forgoing all processed foods.

By this time, however, the years of taking care of the family had taken a toll. "I was unable to work and remained in the house except to give light," says Mary. "I was inconsolable and cried incessantly. I went to all types of physicians." She was finally diagnosed with Hashimoto's hypothyroidism, severe periodontal disease, and numerous environmental sensitivities. Mary had allergies, not the conventional type that produce hives or topical rashes, but sensitivities that caused pain, "brain fog," and hostility. "I was also menopausal and had mitral valve prolapse." Yet her dominant symptoms were still depression, anxiety, and an "I can't do this" type of panic.

Unable to sleep or eat much—due to hot flashes that began every six minutes and lasted for three minutes twenty-four hours a day—she also became very paranoid. The first healing step was hormone replacement, a combination of synthetic estrogen and progesterone (she later switched to natural hormones), which restored her ability to think.

Her dentist for ten years kept saying everything was fine. When she changed to Dr. John Rothchild, who specialized in natural dentistry, phase contrast microbiological analysis showed that she had rampant periodontal disease. Immediate treatment and the removal of silver mercury fillings brought quick mental improvements. "I started to think even more clearly and my depression was lighter."

A friend suggested that she investigate Nambudripad's Allergy Elimination Techniques (NAET). According to founder Devi S. Nambudripad, M.D., D.C., L.Ac., Ph.D., allergic reactions can create a wide range of symptoms, including bipolar disorder, clinical depression, and schizophrenia.[2] Allergic to nearly everything herself, Dr. Nambudripad accidentally discovered how to eliminate her severe allergy to carrots with acupuncture and went on to develop a very effective, noninvasive system for allergy elimination now used by over 7,500 NAET practitioners worldwide.[3]

"I was sensitive to hundreds of things," says Mary, who consulted a local chiropractor trained in NAET. "I was so bad when I first went to see her, I only weighed 145 pounds. My hair was falling out. I was distressed, crying a lot, felt very anxious, and couldn't remember things."

The treatments desensitize patients to one type of substance at a time, after which they refrain from being exposed to it for twenty-five hours. The NAET technique reprograms the nervous system so it will no longer create antibodies, or an allergic reaction, to the substances. "Instead of giving up a particular food or substance for the rest of your life, you can become desensitized to it," explains Mary.

"The really interesting thing I learned after a couple years of treatment was that my body treated a hormone or substance related to my reproductive system, perhaps from the loss of my child, like an invader—triggering an autoimmune response." That required repeated treatments for three years and still needs "reinforcement."

"From there I went on to deal with the prolapsed mitral valve, using a less-than-high-tech approach. My internist says if my heart is pounding out of my chest and I'm dizzy, I need to stop what I'm doing," she says. Deep breathing and specific physical supports return her oxygen levels to normal.

In 2000, with her health vastly improved, Mary began to look for work again. During an interview, one of the three individuals screening her asked a strange question: "If you were in a group of people talking about *recovery* in mental health, how would you relate to them?" Mary replied that she had been a psychiatric nurse for a long time and could relate to all kinds of people. The interviewer stopped her short with "No. How would you relate to people—like *me*—who are in recovery from mental illness?"

This "was the first time I ever heard that someone with any kind of psychiatric condition could recover," says Mary. "After hearing her story, I realized that I had been dealing with my own mental problems which had persisted for decades!" Andrea Schmook was part of a team working for the state of Illinois Office of Consumer Services, which hired Mary for the job she holds today, and became her mentor. "Andrea had all kinds of thing happen to her. She too felt her condition was related to a spiritual crisis, which was a huge validation for me. Although I had never taken psychiatric medications, Andrea did and she eliminated her need for them." (See chapter 11 for Andrea's story.)

"I wanted more information about anything that caused mental problems. Allen is an excellent researcher and found a lot of university studies and information from well-credentialed experts on the Internet, things I never learned in nursing school that are not easy to find in journals." Mary discovered it was true that people could recover from serious psychiatric conditions[4] and there were vastly more and varied causes of the symptoms than are treated by psychiatric clinicians.[5,6]

She began attending Safe Harbor's Non-Pharma conferences in 2003 and went again in 2004 and 2005. "Their information has allowed me to get ahead of my problems," she says. "I began to read medical texts and anything else I could get my hands on about conditions that manifest as mental problems." She learned how to use NAET on different neurotransmitter pathways, taking the information back to her practitioner. "My condition *rapidly* improved after that. I'm now able to partner with my physicians, rather than expecting them to know everything, but the real turning point was meeting someone who had recovered. Today, I know lots of people who have recovered fully from very serious conditions like mine."

About a year after our initial interview, Mary reported that she had begun working with chiropractor Bruce Giffen, N.U.C.C.A., who through x-rays found she had a dislocation of the top vertebrae in her back that put pressure on the spinal cord. Judging by added bone growth to that area, the doctor estimated that the dislocation had occurred around the age of eight, perhaps during one of her fainting spells. After he corrected the dislocation, her constant, internal "stream of negativity," which had persisted and worsened over four decades, suddenly stopped and has not returned. "It's so quiet now in my head!" Mary exclaims. No longer overcome with grief or crying in church, Mary has a renewed interest in understanding the faith in which she was raised.

"I credit and thank God. Because of my persistent spiritual practice, my eyes have been opened. For me, it was a matter of putting my spirit first, then my mind followed, and my body came along for the ride," says Mary. "I've never been better in my entire life. This is a high point. My current job helping the state of Illinois system focus on a *recovery model* for mental health is a dream come true."

The Causes of Allergies

Allergies are abnormal immune reactions to substances that most people find harmless. There are two categories of allergens: environmental (such as pollen, dust, molds, animal dander, chemicals, and cosmetics) and foods. Either can trigger a wide range of symptoms, including depression, autism, schizophrenia, migraines, seizures, arthritis, multiple sclerosis, chronic fatigue, major weight fluctuations, skin and digestive ailments, and heart palpitations.

The primary cause of allergies is a weakened immune system due to hereditary factors, toxic overload, a repetitive diet, or "leaky gut" (explained later). What makes allergies especially complicated, however, is the immune system's highly sophisticated method of determining if something in the body is foreign.

Antigens are unique chemical markers found on the cells of every living organism, from viruses to humans, which form part of its chemical fingerprint. When the body detects a suspicious entity, the immune system compares our antigens to those of the entity to determine if it is "self" or "nonself," an intruder. If it is alien, the immune system produces antibodies that attach themselves to the invader, "tagging" it for destruction.

Antibodies, also known as immunoglobulins, are our cellular defenders. Once an invader is detected, our white blood cells produce billions of immunoglobulin E (IgE) proteins, making a specific variety for each foreign antigen. These bind to mast cells lining blood vessels and basophils, both storage sites for histamine and serotonin. IgE antibodies prompt the mast cell and basophil membranes to "leak," releasing histamine and serotonin into surrounding blood and tissue, injuring the tissue, and causing symptoms known as allergies.[7]

Symptoms may be merely annoying, such as sinus congestion, watery/itchy eyes, and sneezing. Uncomfortable rashes, hives, headaches, digestive upset, and asthma may also stem from allergies. Occasionally, allergic reactions may be life threatening, such as difficulty breathing, heart malfunction, and anaphylactic shock.

The injured tissue uses pain, swelling, redness, and heat—inflammation—to draw the body's repair team. Short-term problems are quickly healed, but when the reaction persists, chronic inflammation is the result. Perpetual inflammation is an underlying cause of medical conditions ending in -itis or -osis, such as arthritis, bronchitis, osteoporosis, multiple sclerosis, and others.

Allergies have long been tied to emotional problems. But because conventional medical wisdom holds that mental illness is not curable, doctors seldom follow this path of inquiry.

There are four categories of allergic reactions, but for simplicity I have grouped them into two—rapid-reaction allergies and delayed-reaction sensitivities (which include autoimmune responses). Rapid reactions indicate conventional allergies that prompt production of IgE antibodies and symptoms within minutes or a few hours of exposure. Delayed reactions involve IgG or IgM antibodies and T-lymphocytes that take twelve to seventy-two hours to manifest, making it difficult to connect them to a specific food (or environmental trigger) except through an elimination diet or blood testing. It is estimated that 95 percent of all food allergies are this delayed type.[8] Prominent among delayed symptoms are chronic fatigue and cerebral allergies that exhibit as mental or emotional disturbances.

How Digestion Is Involved

Ninety-five percent of the body's serotonin is made in the gut. According to Michael Gershon, M.D., author of *The Second Brain*, we have more nerve cells in our intestines (a warehouse for every one of the classes of neurotransmitters found in the brain) than in the entire remainder of our peripheral nervous system.[9]

An association between mental illness and bowel dysfunction was found in several studies in the early 1990s, suggesting a high overlap in these illnesses, ranging from 60 to 94 percent.[10] The connection between the two should come as no surprise. The ability to digest and metabolize is vital to feeding and energizing brain cells. Digestion breaks foods into tiny units that can be absorbed by the body. Metabolism is the internal chemical process by which these units are used for growth, regeneration, internal housecleaning, and energy production.

Enzymes are the catalysts that trigger all biochemical actions in the body. Chewing mixes food with enzyme-rich saliva, which aids in the breakdown of carbohydrates, and enables food to slide easily through the esophagus into the stomach. Stomach muscles blend the mass, called *chum*, with hydrochloric acid and pepsin enzymes that disassemble the amino acid chains in proteins. In the small intestine, bile from the liver (and gallbladder), plus enzymes from the pancreas, further break down fats, fat-soluble vitamins, and proteins. As chum is propelled through the intestines, tiny fully digested food molecules pass through the gut lining into attached blood vessels and are swept away through the bloodstream, which delivers nutrients and calories to all cells, including the brain's.

The lining of a healthy intestine is tight, allowing only completely digested food particles to enter the bloodstream. If digestion is flawed (as with Crohn's disease, irritable bowel syndrome, and celiac disease) and histamine levels are high,[11] the lining becomes inflamed and permeable, allowing large, partially digested molecules to filter through, a condition called "leaky gut."

When the immune system detects any abnormal substance in the body, it begins production of billions of immunoglobulin antibodies to neutralize the invaders and remove them. Undigested food molecules are not "normal" and are interpreted as "alien." Immunoglobulin G (IgG) antibodies are produced to defend against frequently eaten but not properly digested foods that, in turn, trigger allergic symptoms and inflammation. Adequate digestive enzymes are essential for complete breakdown of food molecules.

Primary Digestive Enzymes

Protease	Digests proteins into smaller units, called amino acids
Lipase	With bile (a degreaser) from the gallbladder, breaks down triglycerides (fats) into glycerol (an alcohol) and fatty acids
Amylase	Digests carbohydrates, breaking them into the simple sugars glucose and fructose, fueling all cells
Disaccharidases (also called Carbohydrases)	Digest sugars: sucrose (cane sugar) into glucose and fructose; lactose (milk sugar) into galactose; and maltose (grain sugar) into glucose
Cellulase	Digests the soluble parts of plant fiber into glucose (Only cellulase cannot be made by the body. It is found in raw fruits, vegetables, and whole grains or enzyme supplements.)

The late Dr. Edward Howell, a pioneer in enzyme research, believed that eating raw foods would slow aging because fresh foods contain enzymes the body can use. By providing raw food enzymes for digestion, the body's internal supply is reserved for more vital, metabolic processes. He maintained that the pancreas was never meant to be the sole provider of all digestive enzymes, since early humans and animals primarily consumed raw foods.

Since any temperature above 118 degrees Fahrenheit destroys enzymes, all cooked, pasteurized, canned, and microwaved foods have deactivated, dead enzymes.

Dr. Francis Pottinger was curious about what would happen if mammals were fed primarily denatured, incomplete, or processed foods continuously. His ten-year Pottinger Cats Study concluded in 1983 after following three generations of cats. Two sets were fed only raw milk and raw meat, naturally high in enzymes. Three other sets were fed cooked meat and pasteurized milk, processes that kill enzymes. The cats eating only raw food were disease free and healthy generation after generation. Each succeeding generation of cats fed the processed foods, however, were sicker than the previous one, developing heart disease, cancer, kidney and thyroid disease, tooth loss, arthritis, reduced bone mass, diminished sexual interest, infertility, and such high levels of irritability that they were dangerous to handle.[12]

Fortunately, in 1987 Howard F. Loomis, Jr., D.C., a protégé of Dr. Howell, introduced an option to an all-raw diet: a line of therapeutic plant enzyme supplements available through the Loomis Institute of Enzyme Nutrition in Wisconsin.[13]

Lita Lee, Ph.D., an Oregon enzyme therapist and author of *The Enzyme Cure*, recommends three Loomis enzyme blends for sugar intolerance. Most people in developed countries are sugar intolerant to some degree because we eat so much of it, far exceeding a body's ability to make adequate enzymes for conversion. Sugar intolerance leads to mental and emotional problems, such as panic attacks, depression, insomnia, mood swings, and irritable, aggressive, or violent behavior.[14]

To counter sugar intolerance, Dr. Lee prescribes Chirozyme Pan, a digestive formula containing protease, amylase, lipase, and cellulase with sucrase, lactase, and maltase enzymes. Another formula, called Chirozyme Adr, has the B-complex vitamins plus enzymes and high levels of sucrase. The third enzyme, Chirozyme SvG, combines food sources of vitamins C and E with disaccharidases.[15]

Dr. Lee has found that an inability to digest protein adequately is due to a protease deficiency, which, in turn, leads to anxiety. She recommends Loomis Chirozyme TRMA, a protease blend, to boost the immune system and to alleviate soft tissue inflammation, and panic or anxiety.[16]

In an amazing (and amusingly written) book, *Enzymes for Autism*, author Karen DeFelice, mother of two autistic boys, explains how enzymes support intestinal health and immune function by keeping yeast and bacteria in check. "Bacteria and parasites are made of proteins, viruses have protein coatings or 'films,' and yeasts have outer shells consisting of cellulose and protein. Proteases and cellulases can help break these intruders down."[17] She recommends Peptizyde, for the breakdown of gluten (*not* effective for celiac disease), casein, soy, and other proteins, and HN-Zyme Prime, an all-purpose, broad-spectrum product with a range of enzymes designed to convert all food groups. Both are available from Houston Neutraceuticals.[18]

Like trash collectors, enzymes remove dead tissue, debris, chemicals, and toxins from the body, substances that often interfere with central nervous system functions. If protease enzymes are taken with food, they act on the food first, but taking them *between* meals sends them into the bloodstream to help clear toxins and waste, assisting the liver and the immune system.

Food Cravings and the Brain

Sometimes the foods people long for and eat often are those to which they are allergic because the allergic response impacts opiate receptors, producing "feel good" sensations. When this reaction begins to wear off, the individual wants more of the food, like an addictive drug. One prime example is autistic children who crave milk, although they frequently do not digest it properly and it may aggravate their symptoms.

Another example is the lust for chocolate among people with mood disorders (and many without such disorders). Chocolate is high in copper, so even small amounts contribute to zinc/copper imbalances found in bipolar disorder and violent behavior. Too much chocolate metabolizes to elevated phenylalanine, which contributes to depression or anxiety. Chocolate also contains caffeine, a much-sought-after elixir among tired or depressed people everywhere.

Mental patients with depression also consume large amounts of caffeine (700 mg a day, compared with average American consumption of 255 mg a day), no doubt because it raises levels of serotonin, dopamine, epinephrine, and norepinephrine. Yet caffeine intake has been linked to the degree of mental illness in psychiatric patients: the higher the intake, the more severe the depression.[19, 20]

Several studies have found that caffeine and refined sugar in combination may be even worse, with roughly 50 percent of patients depressed when consuming them together but without symptoms when placed on a caffeine/sucrose-free diet for one week.[21, 22]

Strong food idiosyncrasies or addictions, excessive daily mood swings, perpetual colds or sniffles—all are indicators that what you crave may actually be part of your problem. The most prevalent food allergy triggers are wheat, gluten, milk, corn, chocolate, sugar, and peanuts. According to Peter J. D'Adamo, N.D., tomatoes, potatoes, peppers, and eggplant (all members of the nightshade plant family) generate unhealthy reactions for people with blood types A and O.[23]

How to Diagnose and Eliminate Allergies

Once antibodies are created against a particular food or substance, the immune system sends out more every time it is exposed to that allergen unless specific measures, such as NAET, are taken to "reset" this response. To stop allergies, you must eliminate the cause rather than just suppress the symptoms with antihistamines. This involves establishing a healthy diet, identifying and eliminating foods and substances your body reacts to, healing the gut lining, and then turning off the body's overreaction.

Exposure to environmental allergens that overload the immune system should also be minimized. Stop using pesticides and other synthetic chemicals in your home and garden. Buy dust mite–proof bedcovers and wash them weekly in very hot water. Bathe pets regularly to reduce surface allergens on their bodies, and keep them out of your sleeping areas. Use air filters to reduce pollens and dehumidifiers to dry moisture-laden areas that are prone to mold and mildew.

The cheapest way to identify foods that may be triggering delayed inflammatory sensitivities is through an elimination diet. Simply avoid eating one suspected food for three weeks to allow reactions to clear, and then eat it three times in one day. (Obviously, you should *not* do this with foods to which you have violent allergic reactions.) Observe the symptoms that arise over the next twelve to forty-eight hours—anything from fatigue to headaches, stiffness, anxiety, or depression.

People with leaky gut commonly have dozens of food sensitivities, so an easier approach may be ordering a blood test that measures antibodies. Great Smokies Diagnostic Laboratory[24] is one of a few labs that do IgE and IgG combined food allergy testing. From a vial of blood sent by your doctor, this lab can identify antibody reactions to one hundred foods, for around $200. While this testing does not give all the answers, it offers a quick profile of foods to eliminate as you're healing the gut.

Repairing the digestive tract takes time—for me, after years of undiagnosed celiac disease, about eighteen months. The essential fatty acids that lifted my depression also have anti-inflammatory effects that assist in intestinal healing.

Glutathione, naturally produced by the body, is a crucial antioxidant, immune booster, and detoxifier (see chapter 6). Supplies are diminished by poor diet, pollution, disease, drugs, or aging. Dietary aids that raise glutathione levels include the amino acids glutamine, glycine, glutamic acid, cysteine, and methionine. Whey protein, alpha-lipoic acid, and milk thistle (silymarin) supplements serve the same purpose. Researchers report that glyconutrient supplements increase body levels of glutathione by 50 percent. Researchers in Japan have discovered that the essential glyconutrient N-acetylneuraminic acid blocks release of histamine that causes allergic symptoms.[25]

Supplies of coenzyme Q10, just one of many internally produced antioxidants, may diminish prematurely and need supplementing. Other cofactors in healing the gut are vitamins E and C, together with the minerals zinc, selenium, and magnesium.

Stress plays a big role in allergic reactions, and magnesium helps manage physical and emotional stress. Used by all cells for energy metabolism and protein use, magnesium should be taken in a 1:2 ratio with calcium (i.e., 500 mg magnesium to 1,000 mg calcium) because the body uses them synergistically. Magnesium and calcium should *not* be taken with essential fatty acids, however, because they mutually block absorption. Since calcium and magnesium aid sound sleep, I take mine immediately before retiring.

Beneficial bacteria that populate the intestines, manufacture vitamins, aid digestion, and produce natural antibiotics will be covered in chapter 7. First, let's explore toxins that can open the door to an invasion of yeasts and parasites.

CHAPTER 6

Detoxification: Mercury, Pesticides, and Other Poisons

Imbalances of zinc and copper, two metals naturally found in the body, can bring on the mood swings and rage that often accompany bipolar disorder, according to Dr. William Walsh, a lifelong brain chemistry researcher, specializing in violent behavior. Other contaminants—mercury, lead, arsenic, aluminum, pesticides, and PCBs (polychlorinated biphenyls)—are implicated in central nervous system disorders as well.

Dr. Steven Green, a sixty-year-old bipolar dentist, described with passion how years of exposure to mercury, commonly found in so-called silver dental fillings and other forms, affected his life. Steve's memories of his own volatility and his father's are entwined.

"Anger has colored my whole life," he says. "My father was a dentist with awesome mood swings and perfectionist expectations that made for tense relationships at home and work."

Steve's first recollection of anger was an incident that took place when he was around age three. After he broke something while playing, he remembers his mother saying, "Wait until Dad gets home." Later, whipped by his father with a strap that left long dark bruises down his backside and a hip injury that forever stunted full use of his left leg, he felt betrayed by both parents and "terrified of ever making a mistake again." He and his sister could never risk being funny and "walked on eggshells," constantly cautioned against doing anything that might upset their father.

Steve's exposure to mercury began when his father brought home a "magical" silvery liquid metal, which was sliding around in a little box. His father instructed the kids to "be careful" with it. They played with it until the shiny spheres disappeared into the carpet.

When Steve was fifteen, his father was furious to discover that the boy had massive tooth decay, requiring seventeen mercury amalgam fillings. Once the fillings were in place, Steve's acne worsened, he sniffled with a summer cold that never disappeared, and lymph nodes in his neck and throat were intermittently swollen and tender. "Dad said my body temperature, typically a degree or two below normal, meant that a virus could thrive. My muscles ached for four to five days after weekend sports. Chronic fatigue kept me from endurance events."

Steve limped, had low-back pain, and found awakening in the morning difficult. He frequently had a high-pitched ringing in his ears and complained of headaches. Discovering a small discrepancy in Steve's bite, his father corrected it, ending the headaches.

In spite of a hand tremor, Steve developed excellent hand-eye coordination as a result of constructing many models. He enjoyed the sweet aromatic smells of the glues and paints, which made him feel slightly dizzy while assembling the tiny parts, totally unaware until years later that these poisons synergize in combination.

Meeting his parents' expectations perfectly, Steve was a good student. As high school graduation approached, he had plenty of free time. Housepainting was both a hobby and a source of extra income, so he agreed to paint his father's four-suite professional building inside and out. Paying extra for fungicide in paint (at that time the fungicide was mercury), he worked six to ten hours a day for weeks in a mercurial mist.

The night he graduated from high school, his service club held an all-night party. In the wee hours, underclassmen were throwing all the seniors into the pool. As president, Steve would be last, and he dozed off, awaiting his fate. Awakened and overpowered by six fraternity members, "I suddenly realized the ringleader was the one fellow I did not like. Overtaken by incredible, inappropriate anger, and fueled by its emotional adrenaline surge, I became super-strong and shucked my six attackers. I righteously and mightily swung my right fist at my target's left eye." Fortunately, he missed, breaking the young man's nose instead, knocking him unconscious. Amazingly, his victim apologized the next day.

"What I learned was that I could lose control. I knew I should never own a gun," says Steve. He strove to stay emotionally stable, even avoiding eye contact during conversations, to avoid confrontation at all costs, and perfected an expressive glare meant to be so threatening that it would make people cower and keep their distance.

In dental school, a chuckling junior told Steve he could smell freshmen—they all carried the scent of formaldehyde, another toxin, from handling preserved cadavers in anatomy. As a sophomore, Steve shaped large mercury amalgams with bare fingers, in spite of cursory cautions from instructors. The use of mercury was so common that it was difficult for young students to imagine it could be harmful. Even today, two-thirds of all practicing dentists use mercury amalgam regularly.

Steve married while he was in dental school. "We had a rough time on the honeymoon, not knowing how to cope with my premature ejaculations," he recalls. "But it was my flashes of anger, extreme righteous attitudes, and mood swings over the years that finally took their toll, ending the love."

During the Vietnam War, Steve served in the Navy, working the "amalgam line," in one of twenty-four rooms where young dentists mixed, placed, and carved "silver" mercury amalgams all day long. After a year, with possible orders for Vietnam, he was given seven wartime vaccinations in one hour. "They contained seven subcutaneous doses of thimersol, highly absorbable ethyl mercury." It was the sickest day of his life.

He became dizzy with a high fever and had to quit work early for the first time, collapsing into bed. "My immune system had a new set point for increased inflammatory response. I became plagued by chronic skin rashes, and had increasing aches and fibromyalgia types of pains." The latex gloves used in surgery now triggered contact dermatitis, a massive allergic response that covered his hands and forearms.

Many of the men in Steve's family had heart attacks before age fifty. A routine chest x-ray in his thirties disclosed that Steve had an enlarged heart, an important cardiac risk factor for which the doctor had no answer but a shrug. (When a muscle like the heart is working inefficiently as a result of metabolic poisoning, it becomes larger than expected.) Trying to understand his hereditary predisposition, Steve underwent testing to assess his genetic tendencies.

"Single nucleotide polymorphisms create differences in the way we respond to environmental challenges. Glutathione supports the primary antioxidant and detoxification systems in the body. I have only two of three glutathione genes," he says. This makes him an under-methylator, which intensifies the shortage of glutathione in his body.

"I discovered I was one of 30 percent of the general population who has spina bifida occulta [indicators are a cleft in the chin and a cleft palate], a folic acid weakness that makes us less effective methylators." Methylation (covered in chapter 1), the first step in detoxifying hormones and poisons, helps recycle glutathione. Steve suspects that this is the genetic weakness responsible for his male ancestors' early heart attacks.

"My acetylation is too fast, tending to overload second-phase detoxification. And no gene was present to make interleukin-10, which prevents an excess of inflammation," says Steve. In other words, his genes gave him extremely weak detoxification pathways so his body cannot throw off poisons as effectively as most people. Excessive inflammation over time leads to numerous degenerative diseases.

Steve consulted Andrew Levinson, M.D., in Miami Beach, describing his history of skin rashes, pains, low body temperature, and the aftermath of his seven-vaccination day. Dr. Levinson said, "I think it's the mercury." Steve protested, saying, "But I've been tested for mercury many times in many ways. My hair analysis always shows low levels." However, minerals taken with water worked surprisingly fast, often within ten minutes, to "calm the storm" of Steve's emotions. Heavy-metal symptoms dominate when essential minerals are low because both compete for the same electromagnetic binding sites. Nutritional therapy began to reduce Steve's irritability and pain levels. The doctor ultimately attributed Steve's emotional outbursts to organic affective syndrome, a type of bipolar disorder.

Everyone living in an industrialized society is exposed to multiple toxins, but people who are poor detoxifiers are most harmed because they accumulate the toxins in their tissues. Their systems are so weak at eliminating toxic substances that tests of hair, skin, nail, urine, or blood often do not show toxic levels, even when they exist, because the toxins adhere so tightly to inner molecules they're not excreted. Once in the body, heavy metals occupy sites used by essential minerals, blocking the body's ability to function properly. To determine if mercury, lead, cadmium, or arsenic is present, you must shake the metals loose and get them moving with inherently risky, strong chemicals like DMPS (2, 3-dimercapto-1-propanesulfonic acid).

Dr. Levinson ordered the most predictable test, an intravenous DMPS chelation challenge, preceded by the antioxidant glutathione to minimize the risks. Mercury can cause damage while in the body and when it's dislodged in order to pull it out. Some experts feel DMPS is too dangerous, because rapid chelation can also damage the kidneys. Steve had weekly, then monthly sessions. Six hours after the test, urine was collected, measured for heavy metals, and the data interpreted.

"I was full of mercury. My levels were five times higher than the chart could record." Chelation removes both essential and toxic minerals, so supplementation between sessions is critical. Bipolar people are often erratic and inexplicably perverse. Steve sometimes did not take the essential minerals, even though, as a doctor, he was aware that he should.

After his second chelation, a neighbor excitedly called to say that a man who was a chief adversary in their condominium "wars" was cutting down Steve's trees. Downstairs a short time later, Steve confronted the enemy. "I had a karmic vision—the universe would be totally in balance if there was garbage raining down over this man's head, even if for only one instant." Steve took a partly filled and very smelly garbage bag and swung it hard on top of his adversary's head. Because the bag did not break, he swung it again from the other side. This time the man's fists came up and the bag burst, releasing its contents all over him and the ground.

"I stepped back, both satisfied with and astonished at my actions," says Steve. "The smug look of victory spreading across my enemy's face made me understand the terrible position I had put myself in." Steve was arrested. He was thankful his condominium victim accepted $25,000 and dropped all criminal charges.

Chelation reduces levels of zinc and other beneficial minerals. "Low zinc allows skin infections, makes you smell bad, and increases hypersensitive responses. It causes deficiencies in essential fatty acid function, protein manufacturing, and hormone production. As chelation loosened and circulated mercury so it could be removed, skin infections blossomed and were treated with several courses of intravenous antibiotics. The antibiotics altered my gut flora and function. I suffered my first panic attack and became adrenally exhausted," recalls Steve.

Internal mental changes were most gratifying, however. For the first time, Steve had a more centered, focused, calm feeling inside. He was no longer perpetually late, trying to do too many things at once. "After I acknowledged my own anger while talking with my staff, they began to divulge just how many ways and times they had hidden things from me to avoid triggering my emotional explosions."

Today, Steve's other metal levels are quite low, but mercury is still moderately high. He continues detoxifying and avoiding new toxins. Anger and mood swings are less frequent, he is less aggressive, and he is actually able to make eye contact. His staff says he is a great deal easier to work with. He looks forward to being part of a loving relationship.

Dr. Steven Green is a different dentist now, not only in personality but also in how he practices. He asks patients to have ELISA (enzyme-linked immunoassay) blood tests that use immune responses to show how individuals react to various dental materials. Every body is unique, and a composite material that is perfectly compatible for one patient may be toxic for another. A member of the American Dental Association, Steve attempts to raise awareness of the dangers of old practices from within the organization.

For people wanting more information on mercury amalgam or fluoride dangers, he recommends Web sites for the International Academy of Oral Medicine & Toxicology at www.iaomt.org and Consumers for Dental Choice, a project of the National Institute for Science, Law & Public Policy at www.amalgam.org. To locate environmentally aware dentists nationally, Steve recommends the Holistic Dental Association site at www.holisticdental.org or, for environmental specialists, the American Academy of Environmental Medicine at www.aaem.com.

Mercury and Other Common Toxins

Mercury is used in many products other than fillings. It is a naturally occurring metal that is liquid at room temperature and is found in old thermometers. Because it conducts electricity, it was used in fluorescent lightbulbs, batteries, and other medical equipment now disposed of as hazardous material, but which was in decades past simply hauled to the dump. Mercury has been used in certain medicines, too, so be sure to read labels on antiseptics, mercurochrome, psoriasis ointments, and laxatives.

According to Mark A. Breiner, D.D.S., a Connecticut advocate of mercury-free dentistry, an estimated twenty-four tons of dental mercury are released into U.S. sewers each year by dentists. To give some perspective on just how toxic this refuse is, he says just one molar filling, supposedly "safe" in the mouth, when thrown into a five-acre lake will make all the fish unsafe to eat.

The leading environmental mercury sources today, other than fillings, are coal-burning power plants, waste incinerators, certain pesticides (a category that includes insecticides, fungicides, and algicides), and some grains, sprayed with pesticides. Mercury emitted from power plants and incinerators falls into oceans, lakes, and ponds. It also washes into the sea from farm and lawn pesticide runoff, storm drains, and sewage disposal.

Algae and aquatic microorganisms absorb it. Inorganic mercury is converted to organic methylmercury by microorganisms in sediment. Methylmercury is neurotoxic, meaning it can permanently damage the central nervous system and organs.[1] Big fish eat the small ones and mercury becomes more concentrated at each step up the food chain. Thus, large predatory fish—swordfish, shark, king mackerel, and tilefish—can have levels thousands of times higher than the waters in which they swim.

The level of human consumption of fish correlates with the accumulation of mercury in the body. According to the Environmental Protection Agency, a "safe" level is 0.1 microgram per kilogram of body weight per day, which has been conveniently translated into two servings of seafood a week. According to the Tides Center in Montpelier, Vermont, however, a six-ounce can of tuna contains 0.5 parts per million of mercury and a woman weighing 132 pounds who eats only one can a week is getting too much. The Food & Drug Administration recommends that young children and women of childbearing age avoid tilefish, swordfish, shark, and king mackerel (the top mercury-containing varieties) and limit consumption of all fish to twelve ounces a week.[2]

A peer-reviewed study published in the prestigious journal *NeuroReports* in 2001 by researchers at the University of Calgary Medical School presented the first visual evidence of how mercury disrupts nerve function. Using digital time-lapse photography, Professors Fritz, Lorscheider, Naweed, and Syed, as well as medical student Christopher Leong, recorded the biochemical mechanism. Mercury ions attach to a neuron, causing its microtubules to disassemble, leaving the neuron stripped of its communicating dendrite. Some of these stripped neurons then form aggregates, clumped or tangled together, and the neurons cease to function in a healthy manner. The research showed that mercury induces trademark diagnostic markers in the brain indistinguishable from those seen in Alzheimer's patients and, to date, no other material or metal tested has produced even remotely similar reactions at such low concentrations.[3]

Unfortunately, mercury is not the only substance that contributes to nervous system malfunctions. Lead, arsenic, cadmium, aluminum, pesticides, and PCBs synergistically add to the biochemical load.

Lead is a well-known neurotoxin that produces many psychiatric symptoms: severe depression, overexcitement, restlessness, insomnia, hallucinations, and impairment of memory. Because children's systems are more sensitive than those of adults, children often exhibit learning disabilities or hyperactivity when their body levels of lead or copper are high. Despite years of warnings about the dangers to children from lead poisoning as a result of eating paint chips in older homes and advisories against eating foods on imported, lead-glazed pottery, few homeowners realize that they can be equally adversely affected by inhaling lead particles when sanding old lead-painted surfaces.

For most people, however, lead exposure comes from auto exhaust and coal-fired electric generating power plants. Even people living far from these sources are affected because of the cycle of pollution. Winds carry airborne pollutants thousands of miles from the source. Rain clears them from the air, washing them into reservoirs that serve as sources of drinking water as well as lakes and oceans. When cattle graze in fields near major highways, lead is found in their milk. Lead is also found in colored inks, hair dyes, cosmetics, and cigarette smoke.

Arsenic contributes to anxiety and depression. Sources of arsenic include burning treated wood, coal combustion, insect sprays, pesticides, and eating mussels, oysters, shrimp, chickens fed with arsenic-treated feed, and foods grown in naturally arsenic-rich soils.

Cadmium may cause hyperactivity and, along with lead, contribute to violent or antisocial behavior. It is an airborne industrial metal released by incineration of tires/rubber/plastics or from zinc smelters.

It also is found in batteries and in cigarette smoke, marijuana, galvanized pipes, and rubber backings.[4]

Aluminum, while not a heavy metal, is dangerous in a different way. It sticks to the phosphates that form an active part of DNA (deoxyribonucleic acid), the molecule that gives the body instructions for properly making and replacing cells. Although its presence in the brains of Alzheimer's patients has sparked intense debate about possible sources, what is not debated is that there is no proven method for getting rid of it once it is there.[5] So, avoiding aluminum seems like a wise decision. It's quite simple. Keep aluminum foil out of direct contact with foods, throw out aluminum pans, and stop using aluminum-containing antiperspirants, antacids,[6] and baking powder. No one mentions whether aluminum leaches out of soft drink cans filled with acidic fluids, but on the rare occasions that I drink soda, I choose soda in glass bottles.

Heavy metals bond onto molecules in the body and steal electrons, a process known as oxidation. Lead and mercury are among the worst of a long list of oxidative stressors that we encounter. Because heavy atoms have a stronger pull on electrons, they are more "sticky" and difficult to get rid of, which is why more powerful detoxifying substances, such as DMSA or reduced glutathione, may be needed.[7]

Three Biologically Essential Metals

Copper, zinc, and iron are required by the body in minute amounts but cause problems when levels are too high or when they are not in the proper balance. According to Dr. Walsh at Pfeiffer Treatment Center, imbalances of zinc and copper contribute to rage, violence, obsessive-compulsive disorders, and mania.

Copper can come from dietary sources: seafood, meats, nuts and seeds, soybeans, wheat germ or bran, yeast, gelatin, bone meal, corn oil, margarine, mushrooms, and chocolate (alas). It can be leached out of copper pipes in older homes or unlined copper cookware, or come from birth control pills (estrogen raises copper levels), intrauterine devices, prenatal vitamins, fungicides (in swimming pools or on foods), dental appliances or amalgams, occupational exposure (especially among plumbers and welders), and public drinking water supplies.[8] (Some areas of the United States have naturally occurring copper in the water or copper sulfate may be added to municipal drinking water as a fungicide.) Manganese and zinc supplements are used to reduce copper overload.[9]

Copper imbalances are found with adrenal gland exhaustion because copper oxidizes and destroys the vitamin C required for normal adrenal activity. Congenitally high copper may be due to zinc-deficient mothers. Excess copper can interfere with thyroid activity, lower energy, cause insomnia, and is associated with premenstrual tension and food allergies. Vegetarian proteins are high in copper and low in zinc, and may be a factor in depression.[10]

Zinc in levels that are too low allows copper levels to rise because the two work synergistically and hold each other in check. Zinc deficiency is far more common than excess levels, but it is possible to ingest too much zinc from acidic food stored in galvanized containers or from overindulgence in oysters (the highest food source), seafood, pumpkin, squash, sunflower seeds, mushrooms, milk, or organ meats. Zinc excesses are usually seen, however, when supplementing over 100 mg of zinc per day for several months.

Iron is a component of hemoglobin that carries oxygen to all body cells. Too little causes fatigue, but too much can produce free radical damage to fats in the brain.[11] An estimated 32 million Americans are carriers of a gene for hemochromatosis, a disease of abnormal iron metabolism that causes an overload, although only a small percentage develop the disease.[12] Excess iron can come from drinking water, iron pipes, cookware, welding, or high consumption of organ meats, eggs, blackstrap molasses, clams, oysters, shellfish, and refined foods. Blood ferritin levels should *always* be tested before iron supplements are taken.

Environmental Toxins

In a collaborative study by Mount Sinai School of Medicine in New York and the Environmental Working Group and Commonweal, researchers at two major laboratories found an average of ninety-one industrial compounds, pollutants, and other chemicals in the blood and urine of nine volunteers (who did not work with chemicals on the job or live near an industrial facility). There were a total of 167 chemicals found in the group: 76 cause cancer in humans or animals, 94 are toxic to the brain and nervous system, and 79 cause birth defects or abnormal development. Scientists call such contamination a person's *body burden*.[13]

Researchers in July 2005 found 287 chemicals in the umbilical cord blood of ten newborns, including seven dangerous pesticides, some of which were banned in the United States more than thirty years ago. "Babies don't use any consumer products, they don't work in a factory, and yet they're already starting off with a load of these chemicals," said Dr. Tim Kropp, senior toxicologist for the project.[14]

Environmental toxins commonly found with mental disorders include pesticides and PCBs (polychlorinated biphenyls). Although PCBs were banned in 1977, the damage was already done. One example is General Electric's infamous PCB contamination of New York's Hudson River, which devastated the area's 350-year-old commercial fishery because pollutants on the river bottom are still there thirty years later. According to the National Academy of Sciences, PCBs affect all branches of the immune system and, in cases of prenatal exposure, impact neurological development.[15] PCBs wreak havoc on our cellular systems by producing free radicals that lead to oxidative stress and cell degeneration.

Most pesticides are petroleum-derived and contain xenoestrogens, synthetic substances that unfortunately mimic human hormones by fitting into estrogen receptors in the human body. The known cancer risks from pesticide exposure, according to Marion Moses, M.D., at the Pesticide Education Center in San Francisco, include leukemia, brain cancer, non-Hodgkin's lymphoma, multiple myeloma, and cancers of the pancreas, breast, prostate, kidney/bladder, eye, and colon-rectum. Other long-term effects include elevated risk of infertility, birth defects, Parkinson's disease, and damage to the brain, lungs, kidneys, and liver, and the endocrine, immune, and central nervous systems.

There are less risky ways to have a beautiful lawn or grow delicious produce. See the resources section for information about earth-friendly alternatives for gardening and household cleaning.[16]

How to Safely Detoxify

The first step in getting rid of these poisons—a process called detoxification—is finding an environmentally aware doctor who knows what to test for and how to interpret the data (see Web sites recommended by Dr. Green above).

The most critical organ of detoxification, the liver, was not designed to handle the pollutants that are now part of modern life. It filters the blood to remove toxins, synthesizes and secretes bile with cholesterol and other fat-soluble toxins, and uses enzymes to disassemble unwanted chemicals so the body can dispose of them. The disassembly process is usually referred to as Phase I and Phase II detoxification.

Phase I. Each person has his own mix of around a hundred enzymes with overlapping activities to provide a "fail-safe" detoxification system that oxidizes some chemicals directly while converting others to intermediate forms that are then processed by Phase II enzymes. The oxidized intermediate forms are often more toxic than the original chemicals, so if Phase II systems are not working adequately, these free-radical intermediates hang around and are far more damaging. A side effect of this activity is the production of more free radicals.

For each toxin metabolized, a free radical is generated, and the single most important antioxidant for neutralizing these free radicals in Phase I is glutathione, which is composed of three amino acids: cysteine, glutamic acid, and glycine. Nutrients also required for Phase I detoxification are copper, magnesium, zinc, and vitamin C.[17]

Phase II. Glutathione is also essential for a key process in Phase II detoxification. If the toxic exposure is so high that all the glutathione is used up in Phase I, then Phase II cannot take place, allowing a buildup of toxic intermediates.

There are six Phase II detoxification pathways: glutathione conjugation, amino acid conjugation, methylation, sulfation, sulfoxidation, acetylation, and glucuronidation. Nutrients required for activation of these pathways, and to provide small molecules added to toxins for elimination, are glutathione, vitamin B_6, glycine, S-adenosylmethionine (SAMe), cysteine, methionine, molybdenum, acetyl-CoA, and glucuronic acid.[18]

For people with excessive toxic buildup or liver problems, one of the priorities is to test the phases of detoxification. Sidney Baker, M.D., an autism specialist, describes in *Detoxification and Healing* how caffeine, acetaminophen (Tylenol), and aspirin can be used to show how the body handles other substances too dangerous to administer to test subjects.[19] Each of these products acts like a different class of toxin in the body. By knowing how much is taken of each and measuring the detoxified form later in saliva, urine, or blood, some of the body's efficiency in handling toxins is measured. Great Smokies Diagnostic Laboratory offers materials for this test and a clearly illustrated report of the results.[20]

If you mobilize mercury or other toxins from "safe" storage in body tissues, bringing them out into the bloodstream, and your detoxification capability is not strong enough to finish the job and flush it out in the urine, the toxins can end up in the kidneys, brain, or other organs.[21] They can settle in the lymphatics, especially the breast.

Dr. Baker also recommends the following plan for mercury or lead detoxification. First, have all silver-mercury amalgam dental fillings replaced. (Make sure the dentist uses a rubber "dam" or "cleanup" device to prevent the removed particles from going down your throat.)

Stop eating fish containing high levels of mercury. Limit your consumption of "safe" fish to once or twice a week. Have DMSA testing to determine precise levels of mercury in your body. Depending on the results, begin taking 200 mg DMSA (also called succimer, or a brand called Chemet) three times daily in a three-days-on, eleven-days-off cycle *under a doctor's supervision*, using urinalysis to chart progress. Your own symptoms are the best monitor. Lower the doses if you experience brain fog or distressing symptoms. For a 120-pound person, Dr. Baker suggests 200 mg vitamin C twice daily, 100 mg alpha-lipoic acid three times daily, 200 mg taurine daily, 75 mg reduced glutathione three times daily, 1 mg melatonin at bedtime, plus normal daily doses of zinc (picolinate or citrate), selenium (200 mcg), vitamin E, and vitamin B_6.[22] For lead, he uses the same program with the addition of 1,500 mg of calcium daily.

Far infrared saunas are recommended for reducing your toxic load. Since the skin is the largest organ of elimination, and sweating partially bypasses kidneys, children or patients too weak or elderly to handle DMPS chelation or the extremely high temperatures of regular saunas (180°F to 220°F) can be treated with gentler infrared saunas instead.

Far infrared refers to invisible frequencies of light at the far end of the spectrum that can penetrate the body 1.5 to 3.5 inches. Body tissues selectively absorb these rays as the water in cells react, causing toxins to be dropped into the bloodstream and excreted in sweat, feces, and urine. Temperatures in High Tech Health[23] far infrared saunas are between 100°F and 130°F, causing sweat to contain more toxins and less water. Saunas should be taken under a doctor's supervision, because detoxification can occur too rapidly, causing flulike reactions, and the good minerals sweated out must be replenished.

To avoid toxic overload, watch your diet, reducing alcohol, sugar, saturated or fried fats, and drugs that impede liver function. Avoid eating fish high in heavy metals. Add organic, pesticide-free foods high in fiber, including pears, apples, cruciferous vegetables (broccoli, cabbage), legumes, seeds, nuts, and oat bran. Take high-potency multiple vitamins and balanced amino acids that support detoxification.

Elimination of heavy metals is dependent on the amino acid glutathione, which cannot be synthesized without a sulfur-containing amino acid, N-acetyl-cysteine (NAC). Using NAC, alpha-lipoic acid, and vitamin C together raises intracellular glutathione levels more than just oral glutathione supplements alone, because oral glutathione is poorly absorbed.[24] Also, increase consumption of onions, garlic, and legumes—foods high in sulfur. (Sometimes, poisoned people begin to react to all the sulfur foods.)

Herbs that help detoxify and support the liver can be used in cooking, herbal teas, or taken in supplement form. These include turmeric, Schizandra berries, Thuja, dandelion, nettles, yarrow, milk thistleseed, and lecithin (from soybeans).

Since toxic chemicals are primarily stored in fat tissues, the highest concentrations are in the kidneys and brain. To restore mental health, metals need to be removed, because their presence disrupts central nervous system functions and creates ideal conditions for the overgrowth of a natural yeast, *Candida albicans*, covered in the next chapter.

CHAPTER 7

Halting *Candida albicans* (Yeast) Overgrowth

Elena's health problems started after the birth of her first child. While nursing, she developed mastitis (breast inflammation) and was hospitalized—in the 1950s when new wonder drugs, antibiotics, were proving to be so effective, it was not unusual to be treated with several different antibiotics simultaneously. "The infection retreated all right," she says, "but my body rebelled with diarrhea, malaise, and hives for months. That progressed to rounds of bladder infections, strep throat, and occasional vaginitis for the next few years—always treated with more antibiotics."

After Elena's third child was born, she experienced complete mental and physical exhaustion, diagnosed as postpartum depression. She was hospitalized several times over the next three years.

Although placed on antidepressant medications, she clearly was not getting better. One time she says she "swallowed them all at once in an attempt to end the mental turmoil associated with depression." A series of shock treatments followed. "By now I was convinced I was indeed mentally ill, but I could never understand the reason," she says. Still in a "black hopeless hole of depression," she slashed her wrists and was hospitalized again.

She was finally diagnosed as manic-depressive (today called *bipolar*) and her psychiatrist recommended a new treatment—lithium salts, a natural element—used at the time in Europe and experimentally in the United States but not approved by the FDA until 1974. Elena was required to sign a release holding the psychiatrist blameless in the event that the drug might cause any damage, and it was only administered under strict inpatient supervision. "Finally, I became free of psychiatric hospitals, but not totally free of symptoms," she recalls.

Elena still had severe PMS, short-term depression, severe migraines, food cravings, and emotional outbursts at the least provocation. "I was a woman with two separate minds, indeed. Life was never predictable. It was sane and insane."

Although the lithium salts leveled out her emotional highs and lows with no more extreme depression, "neither was there any joy," says Elena. "Life became an existence, full of anxiety, headaches, and impatience, with a sense of despair about the outcome of my life. I can't say much for the sex life in our marriage. Worse was the continuing bladder incontinence." A gynecologist convinced her all this would be better after a hysterectomy. Without a uterus, there would be no pressure on the bladder. She submitted. Later she learned two things: "The doctor performed an exceptionally high number of hysterectomies and poor bladder function is actually one of the side effects of long-term lithium-salts therapy."

More years went by. Elena slowly became "wracked with daily pain from arthritis in my lower back and sciatica in my leg." Physical therapy and exercise didn't help. A diagnosis of hypoglycemia was added to the roster of her ailments. More bladder infections and strep throat prompted continued use of antibiotics, now mixed with pain medications. "Lithium held me together."

After seventeen years, Elena says, "I wised up! A slow turn of events led to a holistic medical doctor who was familiar with the treatment of systemic *Candida albicans*." Candida is a yeast naturally found in the digestive system that, when it becomes prolific or escapes and colonizes other parts of the body, may cause serious illnesses.

"My senses returned when I realized that *mental illness* is a term used by doctors who do not understand the beastly nature of candida overgrowth and the chemical and hormonal imbalance it causes in certain sensitive people," Elena says. She began a comprehensive program, cutting out all refined sugar, gluten, and most dairy products. She took antifungal medications, acidophilus, vitamins and minerals, did colon cleansing, and took other alternative treatments, including thyroid and adrenal hormone supplements. The therapies brought a profound "stability," and she discontinued lithium in 1986.

"With so many years of reduced vitality—a kind of prison—I began to pursue wellness with a vengeance," says Elena. Breaking ingrained eating patterns and optimizing healthy foods soon "stimulated a new way of viewing the world." She began to exercise and breathe deeply to oxygenate her cells and deliberately changed other daily routines.

"Gradually, I regained my health and my life," she says. "There was little need for drug therapy. No more craziness; no more infections; no stress from unfavorable food, or chemical and environmental exposure."

In the late 1980s, Elena founded the Candida Allergy Support Group, a network to help others "establishing new lifestyle patterns, overcoming conditioning that led us to doubt our well-being." She was invited to join the advisory board of the International Health Foundation, founded by the late Dr. William G. Crook, author of *The Yeast Connection*, and became an articulate and knowledgeable board member.

Elena, now a widow in her mid-seventies, continues to use alternative treatments for all conditions that arise. In 2004, her hair tissue mineral analysis from Analytical Research Labs, Inc.,[1] revealed high copper levels and a low zinc/copper ratio. The report said that high copper is a contributing factor to PMS, urinary tract infections, postpartum depression, as well as various emotional issues.

The report indicates how minerals affect brain function as well as many other body processes: "Our research indicates that individuals exhibiting a copper toxicity are often prone to disorders such as dyslexia. . . . An excess of bio-genic amines [neurotransmitters] results in an increase in brain activity, which can result in anxiety." High levels of copper in the tissues also result in low zinc. Since zinc is required for production of insulin, this interfered with her body's ability to metabolize sugars and simple carbohydrates. The analysis showed that Elena had a low calcium/magnesium ratio, associated with an inability to adequately digest sugars and simple carbohydrates. Low phosphorus levels indicated "inadequate protein synthesis," with the recommendation to increase animal protein intake by 15 percent. The lab also found low levels of chromium, which is needed for fat, protein, and carbohydrate metabolism, and high nickel levels.[2]

Elena used a homeopathic remedy for a year to balance her copper and zinc levels. She has a stainless steel plate in her leg, so she is now taking another homeopathic remedy to reduce the resulting high nickel levels. She uses hydrochloride and digestive enzymes to improve poor digestion, which she attributes to her blood type A. Elena eats according to her blood type and to maintain an alkaline pH in her body—mostly vegetables with small portions of meat and whole grains. She uses no prescription drugs at all. Along with 50 mg of zinc daily, she takes natural forms of adrenal, thyroid, estriol, pregnenolone, and progesterone hormones. Although she used to do yoga, caring for her lawn, her garden with a pond, and her home now provide plenty of physical exercise to oxygenate her cells. For mental exercise, she plays the cello and spends a great deal of time helping others realize that drugs are not the answer to illness.

Intestinal Residents

There are 400–500 different types of bacteria in our digestive systems, roughly 100 trillion living together in either symbiotic or antagonistic relationships. Yet twenty types make up three-quarters of the total, according to Elizabeth Lipski's comprehensive book *Digestive Wellness*. Bacteria manufacture substances that raise or lower our risk of disease, impacting the effectiveness of our immune system, our nutritional use, and our rate of aging.

"Friendly" bacteria are called intestinal flora or probiotics. The two most important bacteria groups are acidophilus (*Lactobacillus acidophilus*), found primarily in the small intestine, and bifidus (*bifidobacterium*), residing mainly in the colon.

Acidophilus prevent overgrowth of disease-causing microbes, such as *Candida albicans*, *E. coli*, *H. pylori*, and *Salmonella*. They aid digestion of lactose and dairy products, improve nutrient absorption, maintain the integrity of the intestinal tract, and help normalize cholesterol levels. Beneficial acidophilus also acidify the intestines, creating a hostile environment for pathogens and yeasts, and preventing vaginal and urinary infections.

Bifidus protect the integrity of our intestinal lining, producing acids that keep microbes from getting a foothold and inhibiting growth of nitrate-producing bacteria. Nitrates are bowel-toxic and can cause cancer. By preventing creation and absorption of toxins by disease-causing bacteria, bifidus ease the liver's workload and enhance immunity. Bifidus also manufacture B-complex vitamins, help regulate bowel movements, and prevent antibiotic-induced diarrhea.[3]

Beneficial bacteria aid protein digestion, freeing amino acids for use, as well as breaking down and rebuilding hormones, all key players in proper brain functioning. Probiotics protect us from heavy metals, pesticides, and other harmful pollutants that impair central nervous system performance. They manufacture many vitamins, including the B-complex vitamins and folic acid, as well as vitamins A and K. Acidophilus and bifidus also secrete lactic acid, enhancing the bioavailability of minerals that require acid for absorption—calcium, copper, iron, magnesium, and manganese.[4]

Symptoms of Yeast Infection

Suspect health problems are yeast-related if you have taken repeated courses of antibiotic drugs, birth control pills, or cortisone drugs. Called "systemic" candidiasis when it has escaped the gut and made itself at home in other parts of the body, this colonization can trigger a wide range of symptoms: behavior and learning problems, such as hyperactivity, poor memory, and aggressive or inappropriate behavior; emotional changes like rapid mood swings, depression, irritability, or anger; loss of sexual interest; muscle aches, cramps, and fatigue; sugar cravings; numerous allergic reactions; chemical sensitivity; kidney and bladder infections, or vaginal or rectal itching or discharge; white patches in the mouth or a rash akin to diaper rash; digestive disturbances such as diarrhea, constipation, bloating, irritable bowel syndrome, nausea, and cramps; or feeling "sick all over" without a known cause.[5]

Dr. Leon Chaitow in *Fibromyalgia Syndrome* cites one practitioner's report that 90 percent of her patients with fibromyalgia had yeast infections.[6]

One of my favorite wellness doctor/authors, Julian Whitaker, M.D., in *Dr. Whitaker's Guide to Natural Healing*, includes a three-page candida questionnaire to help you determine if the yeast is causing your illness. Because candida is resistant to both drugs and alternative treatments, he proposes a comprehensive approach: following an anticandida diet, improving digestion, detoxifying, boosting the immune system, and taking nutritional and herbal substances to kill off the organism.[7]

The late William G. Crook, M.D., a pediatrician and author of *The Yeast Connection* and *Help for the Hyperactive Child*, wrote that children most likely to have candida overgrowth are those given repeated antibiotics for ear or other infections. Once the yeast dominates, digestive flora become imbalanced, the immune system becomes weakened, and "leaky gut" brings increasing allergies and triggers depression, irritability, and/or hyperactivity. Dr. Crook recommended a special sugar-free diet and oral antiyeast medication instead of the popular drug Ritalin. Although some doctors prescribe Diflucan, that alone may not work because the yeast is resistant and quick to repopulate. To control yeast overgrowth and restore normal bacteria in the intestinal tract, Dr. Crook used nonprescription therapies: caprylic acid, probiotics, citrus seed extracts (such as Paracan 144, Paramicrocidin, and Citricidal), garlic cloves and/or Kyolic, and the herbal product Mathake (*Terminalia catappa*). Yeast-free, sugar-free, color-free nutritional supplements are also very important, as are essential fatty acids and bioflavonols, grapeseed extract, and Pycnogenol™ (pine bark extract).[8]

Certain foods feed the yeast. The list is long: sugar and sugary foods; packaged foods; most condiments and sauces; dried fruit and fruit juices; refined grains or carbohydrates; fermented and aged dairy products; processed, aged, cured, and/or smoked meats or fish; peanuts and pistachio nuts (due to high mold content); sweetened chocolate; alcoholic and caffeine-containing drinks; and all yeast-containing foods, such as breads, cheeses, vinegars, soy sauce, cider, or mushrooms. Check all supplements to be certain they are yeast-free.[9]

Nearly eighty different toxins are produced by yeast overgrowth. They make you chronically tired, interfere with vitamin and mineral absorption, and can affect body hormones and alter nerve transmission, befuddling the brain. Toxic overload taxes the immune system too, which is why people with candida sometimes feel as if they are allergic to everything. Because of this oversensitivity to everyday chemicals (perfumes, cleaning products, paints, pesticides, insecticides, tobacco smoke, diesel fumes, etc.), physical exposure should be limited whenever possible.

Over-the-counter candida-fighting products and probiotics are readily available at health food stores. Do not mistakenly believe you can replenish the good bacteria in your gut simply by eating yogurt containing live cultures. One doctor said I would have to eat forty pounds of yogurt a day to get enough good bacteria. The packages of probiotics provided by my naturopath bore this out—they contained 3 *billion* bacteria in each dose.

Also, be aware that candida treatments can cause die-off reaction, a flulike syndrome lasting a day or more as the dying bacteria give off toxins. As these toxins are eliminated from the body, symptoms will clear up. However, this yeast is resilient and quick to repopulate, so rebalancing an excess of candida may be difficult. No single protocol works for everyone because of individual genetic and metabolic differences. One successful protocol is included in appendix B. Find a doctor experienced in treating this problem and discuss the plan with him or her.

Self-Administered Brain Disruptors

Alcohol, caffeine, tobacco, sugar, chocolate, artificial sweeteners, monosodium glutamate, and fluoride are all substances that disrupt brain function. Abuse of any of the first four is a red flag that undiagnosed depression or other mental disorders may be present. Substance abusers may be unconsciously self-medicating, trying to lift their spirits or energy, but the fix is always temporary and actually contributes to the down cycle.

"Most addicts are *born* with subnormal moods," says Julia Ross, M.A., who has worked in and directed addiction-recovery programs for over twenty-five years in the San Francisco Bay Area (and helped the women whose stories are told in chapters 8 and 10). If you and other family members have severe alcohol, drug, and/or food addictions, you may have inherited genetic deficiencies in the brain's ability to produce natural mood boosters.[10]

Alcohol is a well-documented depressant. Consumption temporarily increases brain serotonin turnover, improving mood, but results in additional neurotransmitter depletion. So, an alcoholic feels better after a drink but is more depressed than ever the next day.[11] According to Ross, 90 percent of alcoholics who try to quit using twelve-step programs and standard psychological approaches fail because these do not address the primary cause of addiction, which is *physical.* Specific solutions for addictions are beyond the scope of this book, but you may learn more by reading Ross's books, *The Diet Cure* and *The Mood Cure*, and by contacting her clinic, Recovery Systems, in Mill Valley, California, for addiction therapy (see Resources).[12]

Caffeine. A popular stimulant found in coffee, tea, soft drinks, chocolate, and cocoa, caffeine is also used in Excedrin, Anacin, and many other medicines. In one study of healthy college students, moderate and high coffee drinkers scored higher on a depression scale than low users—and it apparently didn't help their concentration, because they also had lower academic performance.[13] People prone to depression or anxiety tend to be especially sensitive to caffeine. In one study of psychiatric patients, the higher the intake of caffeine, the more severe their depression.[14]

Tobacco. Nicotine stimulates adrenal hormone secretions, including cortisol. Cortisol activates tryptophan oxygenase, resulting in less tryptophan being sent to the brain. Since serotonin production depends on tryptophan, smoking reduces levels of this "feel good" neurotransmitter. Cortisol also "down-regulates" serotonin receptors, making them less sensitive to what little is available. Tobacco lowers vitamin C levels, and low vitamin C in the brain can result in depression or hysteria.[15]

Sugar. Refined sugar is a carbohydrate that does not contain the protein, vitamins, or minerals necessary for its own metabolism (while fruits and natural sugars usually do), so it diverts nutrients, especially the brain-critical B-vitamins, from other parts of the body to do the job. Excessive sugar consumption can lead to an imbalance of calcium and phosphorus. It makes the digestive system work harder to prevent too much sugar from entering the bloodstream all at once. The pancreas has to increase production of insulin to process the sugar, which takes away energy from the immune system and contributes to hypoglycemia (see chapter 3), with resulting mood swings.

Yet, people with brain chemistry disorders *crave* sweets and refined starchy carbohydrates that quickly convert to glucose, giving an almost instantaneous sugar high. Perpetual sugar or carbohydrate cravings may be a signal of low serotonin. Although serotonin is made from tryptophan, an amino acid found in protein, serotonin-releasing brain neurons are unique because the amount of the neurotransmitter released depends on the ratio of insulin and tryptophan in the blood. So eating protein alone, without carbohydrates, may not trigger sufficient serotonin release to meet the body's needs.[16]

The best way to tame cravings, and reduce total sugar intake, lies in balanced meals or snacks containing carbohydrates and protein together. If cravings persist, take vitamins, minerals (especially chromium and magnesium), and specific amino acids. Julia Ross recommends taking 150 mg of 5-HTP three times a day between meals for sugar and carbohydrate cravings. To raise energy levels or to boost concentration, take 500–1,000 mg of tyrosine upon arising and midmorning. To calm yourself, take 100–500 mg of GABA, as needed. To ease hypersensitivity and promote emotional comfort, take 500–1,000 mg of DLPA, a combination of D- and L- forms of the amino acid phenylalanine, on arising and midmorning.[17] Once you are getting the nutrients your brain needs, cravings should cease, letting you effortlessly stop using brain disruptors.

Artificial Sweeteners. In an attempt to cut back on sugar and calories, many people turn to calorie-free artificial sweeteners, the most popular of which is aspartame (NutraSweet®, Equal®, and Spoonful®). Aspartame is made from amino acids, which sounds totally safe. But aspartame has three components: the amino acids phenylalanine and aspartic acid, and methanol. By 1988, aspartame had the longest list of complaints the FDA (Food and Drug Administration) had ever received—over three thousand. People complained of symptoms from mild depression and suicidal depression to seizures, memory loss, and blurred vision, as well as rashes, headaches, nausea, vertigo, and insomnia.[18]

In the body, aspartame is broken down into toxic formaldehyde, formic acid, and methanol. Methanol, also known as methyl alcohol or wood alcohol, is poisonous even in modest amounts. When you consider that aspartame is found in cereals, gum, yogurt, frozen desserts, laxatives, multivitamins, pharmaceuticals, toppings, tabletop sweeteners, and hundreds of beverages, a person's daily consumption may be anything but modest.

In the brain, one of aspartame's components, phenylalanine, is converted into the stimulating neurotransmitters tyrosine, dopamine, norepinephrine, and epinephrine. Aspartic acid and phenylalanine both compete with and beat out tryptophan (the precursor to serotonin). So if you are already low in serotonin, you certainly should not be drinking diet sodas or artificially sweetened coffee that contains both aspartame and caffeine.[19] Instead, drink flavored waters or herbal teas.

Ralph Walton, M.D., professor and chairman of the Department of Psychiatry at Northeastern Ohio Universities College of Medicine, says, "We have known for years that when aspartame is ingested with a carbohydrate-rich meal, the usual physiologic increase in tryptophan is blocked, while brain phenylalanine and tyrosine concentrations are increased." He believes that these changes alter the fragile balance in the brain, causing a "profound effect on mood and cognition," including loss of memory.[20] Try remembering that before ordering a diet soda with fries.

Monosodium Glutamate (MSG). Glutamic acid is an amino acid that excites and even kills brain cells in laboratory animals. Commonly used as a salt, known as glutamate, glutamic acid comes in two forms: one bound to protein and one free of protein, MSG. The free form is often added as a flavor enhancer because it affects the way the brain senses flavors, suppressing bitterness and sourness. In the food industry, this means increased profits, making it a common additive in thousands of processed foods. The problem is you don't always know it is present because of inadequate labeling laws. If a product contains 99 percent protein-free glutamic acid, it is called monosodium glutamate (MSG) and must be labeled that way. However, free glutamate in lesser strengths may be included in processed foods under dozens of different names (see box).

According to Skye Weintraub, N.D., in *Allergies and Holistic Healing*, the reason some people have allergic reactions to glutamic acid while others do not is unclear, but to many the free form is definitely harmful. Free glutamic acid can cause mild intoxication, flushing, and confusion. It adds to the allergic load, increasing sensitivities to numerous chemicals and other substances. Often the reaction depends on the dose, but with people who do not metabolize MSG effectively, even tiny amounts act like a poison.

If the blood-brain barrier has been damaged by head trauma, stroke, diabetes, hypoglycemia, or aging, MSG can pass through, impacting the brain like a drug. Dr. Weintraub lists more than thirty-six symptoms that may stem from ingesting free glutamate. Those relating to the brain include anxiety attacks, disorientation, mood swings, ADHD, depression, hyperactivity, drowsiness, and seizures.[21] Obviously, it is a food additive that should be avoided.

Ingredients That Always Contain MSG

Monosodium glutamate (MSG)

Glutamate

Calcium caseinate

Yeast food

Autolyzed yeast

Gelatin

Ingredients That Often Contain MSG

Bouillon, broths

Malt extract, malt flavoring, maltodextrin, barley malt

Whey protein, soy protein, soy protein isolate, processed proteins

Pectin

Corn starch

Carrageenan

Soy sauce

Citric acid

"Natural flavors or flavorings" (chicken, pork, beef, etc.)

"Seasonings"

Protease enzymes, enzymes, modified enzymes

Powdered milk, anything ultrapasteurized

Unexpected Sources of MSG

Salad dressings

Cheese

Ice cream

Beverages

Frozen meats

Reduced-fat milk

Cookies

Candy

Chewing gum

Packaged and restaurant soups

Asian restaurant foods

Vitamin-enriched foods

Supplements, especially minerals

Medications

IV medications

Vaccines

Source: J. Samuels, "MSG—Dangers & Deceptions," The Price-Pottinger Nutrition Foundation, reported at www.becomehealthynow.com.

Chocolate. Many children with mood disorders are highly allergic to chocolate. Lots of adults are both addicted to and sensitive to it. I am. A single candy bar often lowered my immunity so quickly that I would come down with whatever bug was going around within twenty-four hours. A one-inch-square, wafer-thin piece of chocolate lowered my body temperature by one degree overnight. Yet, chocolate always made me feel great emotionally and, because of my celiac disease, it was one dessert I could eat.

Why is this dark decadence so hard to resist? Chocolate is high in phenylethylamine (PEA), an amphetamine-like stimulant that, along with sugar, is a highly addictive mood elevator, and PEA levels in depressed patients are always low.[22] Cocoa powder contains more magnesium than any other food, so one might also be a "chocoholic" because the body is signaling for more magnesium. (Sorry, cocoa is *not* the best way to replenish magnesium. Increase consumption of whole grains and beans instead.) Also, excessive sugar needed to sweeten chocolate leaches calcium from bones, ultimately creating a greater calcium/magnesium imbalance.

Fluoride. There are two types of fluoride: calcium fluoride, the type found in nature, and sodium fluoride, which is added to drinking water. Fluoridation of U.S. public water supplies began in 1945 as a means of reducing tooth decay, based on research by H. Trendley Dean, D.D.S., with data he later admitted in court was invalid.

Although 10 percent of fluoride in adults is deposited in the bones, studies have since shown a correlation between higher fluoride intake and a decrease in bone mass and strength over time.[23] In 1975, John Yiamouyiannis, M.D., and Dean Burk, M.D., compared ten large U.S. cities that fluoridated their water with ten cities that did not and discovered a link between fluoride and a 10 percent increase in cancer deaths. Congress ordered studies that confirmed that fluoride added to water causes cancer in laboratory animals, but no action was taken. Fluoride and chlorine are both associated with reduced levels of T_4, the thyroid hormone, perhaps because the two substances are chemically similar to thyroid-vital iodine, so they may displace it in the body.[24, 25, 26]

Common in this country's drinking water, fluoride has been banned in Austria, Denmark, France, Greece, Italy, Luxembourg, the Netherlands, Norway, and Spain.

People with depression, bipolar disorder, or any psychological disorder should completely avoid all of the above brain disruptors.

CHAPTER 8

Eliminating Parasite Infestations

In Japan on Halloween in 1988, after a typical day of trying not to eat anything but finally giving in and overeating until her stomach was distended, Vickie went into the bathroom, put a finger down her throat, and threw up. Known as "purging," it was the first time she had done such a thing and the beginning of a nightmare.

A couple months earlier, twenty-two-year-old Vickie went to Osaka to work as a housekeeper and cook for a wealthy family who owned an American restaurant. Five foot six inches tall, always a healthy eater but never weight obsessed, she began overeating shortly after she arrived, gaining thirty-five pounds in two months. "Looking back," she says, "I suspect I had always been mildly depressed, even from the time I was young. But how do you label that? You don't know." In Japan, Vickie simply thought the depression and desperation stemmed from the fact that her clothes no longer fit and that she was suddenly obsessed with food.

Alone all day, Vickie tried to avoid eating by staying busy in the four-story house. "We didn't wear shoes indoors, so it was an extremely clean house to begin with. I never cleaned a dirty floor; I kept cleaning clean floors," she says with a laugh. Unable to drive, she walked to the market daily, carrying back whatever she would prepare for dinner: mushroom cheeseburgers, big casseroles, and other American favorites the family loved.

The walk took her past Kentucky Fried Chicken and a favorite donut shop. In spite of her resolutions, she always stopped. "Basically, I would overeat anything I could get my hands on," she says, "and I didn't know why. No amount of food satisfied me. I felt gluttonous and very self-critical. It became intolerable.

"After I purged the first time, I cried and cried, felt guilty, and swore to myself I'd never do it again. But I couldn't resist. My urge to overeat stayed just as strong, but I had found a solution—to throw it up afterward.

"If I started putting any food in my mouth, I couldn't stop. I'd open a bag of fried, sweetened banana chips, thinking I would eat a handful, and I would finish the whole bag and just be sick with myself," she says. "Then it was like, if I've eaten that much, I might as well keep going. So I would go on to popcorn or whatever was around that I could eat without being noticed."

After six months, she returned to the United States, but the urge to overeat continued unabated. College was too difficult, given her compulsion, so she dropped out. "I planned my day around when and where I was going to eat and throw up.

"All my relationships suffered," Vickie recalls. "You know when you're madly, crazy in love, and the person goes away and you just long for him, and dream of him, and can't stop thinking about him. I was like that for food." She didn't go out to dinner with girlfriends if they were going to a movie afterward, because she needed to find a private place to purge.

Vickie loved cocaine the moment the effects hit her brain. "It was the first time in years that I had not had food on my mind constantly, because the stimulant takes away the urge to eat. So it was absolute heaven to me. I became hooked pretty quickly." The pounds started coming off, too, until her weight fell below one hundred pounds, bringing compliments that shored up her low self-esteem.

"Eventually, the drugs ran out and the people ran out. Coming off stimulants is horrific—the depression is unbelievable. I discovered drinking." Alcohol took the edge off her drug cravings. Far from the ideal solution, it simply introduced a new compulsion. "Whenever I drank, I couldn't stop myself. I would drink to oblivion almost every day."

Somehow, Vickie managed to work at restaurants, either as a hostess or a cashier, through years of drug addiction and alcoholism. After work, she and her boyfriend would drink in bars until closing time. Frequently, she blacked out, unable to recall what happened or where her car might be. One day she awoke, her whole body in pain, a tooth loose, and she felt "like I might die." Her boyfriend described how she had instigated a fight with another woman and the brawl that ensued. "It was horrible, low-life behavior, that's painful for me to even tell you now," she says quietly.

After more days of straight vodka, "no ice, no mixer, no little olives—I drank it like water," Vickie lay in bed contemplating suicide. The only thing in the house she could use was alcohol. She tried to figure out if she had enough alcohol to kill herself or if it would just make her sicker. "I knew I couldn't wake up the next morning and continue to drink. But I also knew there was no way I could wake up and not drink."

The next morning she started calling treatment centers, trying to get in. Some wanted to put her on a waiting list, but she knew if she didn't get in somewhere that day, she might not make it to the next. Finally, one center agreed to admit her immediately. A friend drove her to "a no-frills, hard-core, bottom-of-the-barrel, drug and alcohol rehab" center for a seven-day detoxification and a twenty-eight-day rehabilitation program.

"It absolutely changed my life," Vickie says. "I never drank again after that. It gave me a whole new beginning." Expecting to be the only twenty-seven-year-old female in a room full of men, she was shocked to find herself with people of all sexes and ages, from all walks of life. "The problem was, through the entire thirty-five days, I continued to binge and purge." After completing the program, she went to meetings, continuing her alcohol recovery, but was still bulimic.

Bulimia was far more difficult when she was sober. "I would go to twelve-step meetings, share all the beautiful things that had begun happening, and begin to feel a connection to a higher power, but I still felt like I was lying," Vickie says, "since I was still purging."

Her best friend hired her as a nanny, offering a lovely private room as payment. "I think that made me realize how miserable I was, being around such a beautiful, healthy family, seeing how they lived. I would be bingeing on pizza in my room and hear them laughing in the kitchen together," she recalls with a break in her voice.

Sitting in the friend's kitchen, chatting with her one day, Vickie came across an article in the Whole Foods Market magazine about Julia Ross's treatment of eating disorders at Recovery Systems in Mill Valley, California, a suburb of San Francisco. It was brief, but Julia's description of the food addict's compulsion was "the very first time I had ever read anything by anyone that I felt understood my predicament."

Vickie took the magazine back to her room, because bulimia was a disgusting secret she had never acknowledged even to her best friend. She made an appointment and flew to San Francisco.

"Julia's clinic sent me paperwork ahead of time: food/mood charts, a diary of what I was eating, and tons of intake questionnaires. The initial appointment lasted four hours." Vickie went on a high-protein, low-carbohydrate meal plan. She had to eat at least four ounces of protein three times a day at meals, plus protein snacks, like nuts and seeds.

Two things made an immediate difference. "I stopped eating all the foods that my body didn't tolerate—wheat and gluten products—the things that I wanted to binge on most." She also stopped eating all other addictive foods, caffeine and sugar (including artificial sweeteners), and lived for months on a diet of meat, vegetables, nuts, seeds, and small amounts of fruit.

Tests showed that Vickie had an overgrowth of the yeast *Candida albicans*, so she was put on an antiyeast protocol too.

"I can't remember all the supplements I was taking. Lots of amino acids from the second I got up in the morning until I went to bed at night. I was on L-tryptophan to boost my serotonin. I did L-glutamine, D-L-phenylalanine, and L-tyrosine," she says. Her thyroid was checked and found to be underactive, so she began taking thyroid medication. She was instructed to eat plenty of good fats—grapeseed oil, olive oil, omega oils, nuts, and a little butter in cooking, but no margarine, hydrogenated oils, or processed oils. Aloe vera juice was very soothing to her gut. She took acidophilus and other probiotics as well. "I was on so many pills I completely freaked out. I said, 'Julia, I'm an addict—you're telling me to take thirty pills a day.' Julia said, 'Vickie, they're the building blocks of protein! They're natural—you're not going to feel any of it as if they were drugs.' She was right, of course."

Vickie never purged again, which is unusual with severe eating disorders, and her underlying depression is gone. "I think part of the key was pulling me off all the foods that I reacted to and wanted to binge on, giving my brain a chance to repair itself with all the aminos."

After about five months, Vickie called Julia in tears, saying, "I'm not purging and I'm not eating bread and pasta or anything like that, but I *want to* so bad that it makes me cry." Julia told Vickie something was still wrong—that she should be free of the compulsion by now. She ordered stool sampling, checking for parasites. The results showed Vickie was yeast-free, which was good, but that she had a high concentration of the parasite *Blastocystic hominis*.

"Being the skeptic that I am, and being aware of the placebo effect, I called the lab guy instead of Julia. He didn't have my diagnosis, all he had was my name and the ID number of the sample, so he didn't know I was bulimic." Vickie simply told the man she wanted to verify her results and understand what they meant. A zero concentration meant no parasites; a four meant the highest concentration. Vickie had a level three of *Blastocystic hominis*. "I asked, 'What is this and what does it do?' He said, 'Do you crave starch and fat?' I said, 'Every waking minute.' He said, 'This parasite craves starch and fats. If you get rid of it, then your cravings will go away.'

"I was given two options. Either take antibiotics or go a natural route, neither of which was guaranteed to work, because the guy at the lab said they [*Blastocystic hominis*] are really hard to get rid of." Vickie chose natural remedies.

She started the parasite protocol (created by Timothy Kuss, M.A.,

C.N.C., of Infinity Health, and included in appendix C), then simply went on with life. One day, "I realized that I didn't want to cry when I walked down the bread aisle anymore. In the freezer section by the ice cream, I wasn't distracted. I didn't care. Suddenly, I had freedom. The obsession was gone."

Without depression, food obsessions, or addictions, Vickie enrolled at a community college, then transferred to a university and graduated with a bachelor's degree in psychology with honors. She has completed graduate school and is presently working on a thesis about nondrug treatments for mental disorders and the role of nutrition in mental illness.

No longer needing a lot of amino acids now that healing is complete, this slim, dark-haired, energetic young woman simply sticks to a healthy diet, taking basic vitamin and mineral supplements, thyroid medication, and 5-HTP for PMS or whenever she starts feeling blue.

Parasites

The word *parasite* generally refers to any organism that lives off another host, but in the medical context, it refers specifically to protozoa (single-cell organisms), arthropods (insects), and worms that invade and feed off the host, often causing harm. Although they have evolved with human beings for as long as anyone can tell, parasites in the body appear to have no beneficial purpose. They do, however, contribute to a variety of major illnesses: psychiatric disorders, Crohn's disease, ulcerative colitis, arthritis, rheumatoid symptoms, chronic fatigue, Epstein-Barr virus, as well as AIDS.[1]

The protocol included in appendix C is designed to combat seven different protozoas, including *Blastocystic hominis*, which has been linked to acute and chronic illness. Another, *Giardia lamblia*, is a virulent parasite, found in contaminated water, that is often the source of traveler's diarrhea. *Entamoeba histolytica* can cause dysentery and injure the liver and lungs. *Dientamoeba fragilus* is associated with diarrhea, abdominal pains, itching around the anus, and loose stools. *Cryptosporidium* is a threat to people with already compromised immunity.[2]

Insect parasites (lice, mites, ticks, and fleas) carry other, smaller infectious organisms, such as *Borrelia burgdorferi*, the spirochete-shaped parasite that causes Lyme disease, and *Yersinia pestis*, which causes bubonic plague. Worm-type parasites include pinworms, roundworms, tapeworms, *Trichinia spiralis*, hookworms, Guinea worms, and filarial (threadlike worms in the blood and tissues).

Frank Strick, clinical research director of the Research Institute for Infectious Mental Illness, says people with chronic candida yeast infections often have both parasitic infestations and viruses that create an obstacle to long-term cures.

The parasite *Toxoplasma gondii* (usually spread to humans from cats) is known to alter behavior and neurotransmitter function. Says Strick, "Since 1953, eighteen out of nineteen studies of *T. gondii* antibodies in persons with schizophrenia and other severe psychiatric disorders have reported a higher percentage of *T. gondii* antibodies in affected persons."[3] (Tests typically measure antibodies produced by the body in reaction to invaders instead of the difficult-to-locate pathogens themselves.)

A 2005 study in the *American Journal of Psychiatry* stated, "Toxoplasmosis is known to adversely affect fetal brain development," and found that expectant mothers with high levels of antibodies to this parasite during pregnancy (meaning they had had greater exposure) were more than twice as likely to have schizophrenic children.[4] Another study showed that the antipsychotic drug Haldol and the mood stabilizer valproic acid (used for schizophrenia and bipolar disorder) inhibit toxoplasma growth in laboratory tests, suggesting that their antiparasitic action may actually be what reduces psychiatric symptoms.[5]

In parasite infections that can be seen through imaging techniques (that is, in cases where the brain is directly invaded)—such as neurocysticercosis (caused by a tapeworm)—depression and psychosis were found 65 percent of the time. With other less visible forms, like giardiasis, ascaris (roundworm), and trichinae (from eating undercooked pork), documentation is more difficult, usually coming only when the hidden infection is treated for other reasons and psychiatric symptoms disappear.[6]

The brain's function is impaired by parasites because they live off their host, stealing nutrients, interfering with enzyme and immune function, and releasing massive amounts of toxins as waste products. These toxins, at high levels, can lead to blackouts, muscular and skeletal pain, menstrual irregularities, and wide swings in blood sugar levels and mood.

Viruses (submicroscopic parasites) are also prime suspects in psychiatric symptoms. People infected with HIV (human immunodeficiency virus) have shown a heightened risk of developing mood disorders.[7] Researchers at Tulane University School of Medicine found that 52 percent of patients suffering from schizophrenia and bipolar disorders had retroviral exposure (that is, exposure to a group of viruses that contain RNA and reverse transcriptase), compared to 25 percent of those without psychiatric symptoms.[8] Another study found retroviruses "weakly" correlated to schizophrenia and bipolar disorder, but noted that they "may be influenced by the individual genetic background."[9]

German researchers made cultures of an animal *borna* virus— obtained from people with depression or manic-depression—and found antibodies against the virus in other patients. "We have strong evidence that this virus is involved in human central nervous system disorders," said Dr. Hanns Ludwig, professor of virology at Free University in Berlin. Half the three hundred depressed patients they studied had borna antibodies, compared to 1 percent of controls.[10] A Japanese study exploring this connection in 2005 found borna virus antibodies in 4 percent of control subjects, 22 percent of patients with schizophrenia, and 27 percent of those with mood disorders.[11]

Contracting Parasites

It is easier to contract parasites than you might think. Raw fish, shell-fish, and meats are common sources. Since Vickie ate sushi only once during her stay in Japan, she probably got her parasite from inadequately washed fruits or vegetables.

Protozoa parasites are most often found in feces-contaminated water—in rivers, streams, groundwater wells, or overcrowded and temporary communities, such as refugee camps and institutions. Giardia is a highly contagious variety carried by cats, dogs, other animals, or people, that can be transferred by simply petting or touching the carrier and then touching your mouth. Day-care centers are a breeding ground for parasites, as are pediatric and dental clinics. Pinworms are the most common variety caught by children that spread throughout the family.

According to Peter J. D'Adamo, N.D., people with blood types A and AB are at higher risk for contracting parasitic infections because they have naturally low stomach acid, due to their genetic makeup.[12] Hydrochloric acid in the stomach helps kill germs and parasites. Without enough of it, digestion is weak and the "bugs" survive, taking up residence in the body. Since children's systems are less well developed, they are more susceptible.

Travelers pick up parasites and may suffer minor symptoms for years before anyone thinks to do laboratory analysis of a stool sample. With the influx of foods grown around the world, and the popularity of uncooked or partially cooked sushi and sashimi, everyone's exposure is increased.

Avoiding Parasites

Prevention includes cleaning all raw fruits or vegetables that will be eaten uncooked (see below) and eliminating unpasteurized dairy products, raw meat, poultry, or seafood from your diet.

Food Preparation. Use a separate cutting board for meats and vegetables. Wash your hands and all utensils thoroughly *with soap* after handling raw meat or using the bathroom. Wash vegetables and fruit thoroughly, particularly salad items. Plunge fresh produce into a gallon of water to which is added a few drops of grapefruit seed extract *or* one tablespoon of apple cider vinegar and one tablespoon of hydrogen peroxide. Soak for twenty minutes, rinse, and soak in fresh water ten minutes before serving or refrigerating. While traveling, do not eat at unsanitary places. If that is unavoidable, eat only hot, cooked foods, nothing raw (especially salads, ice, milk, or ice cream).

Water. Don't drink from streams or rivers, even if they look crystal clear. If your home's water source is a well, have the water tested by a private laboratory. When traveling, drink only bottled water, checking where it was bottled and making sure the seal is not broken. (In some areas, bottles are refilled from a local tap.) Be sure to avoid eating salads and other raw foods that may have been washed in contaminated water. Also be cautious about swimming in lakes or ponds when traveling. If you're swimming in a public pool, ask where the water comes from and how it is treated. (I was on a lovely cruise in Egypt that featured filtered water throughout the ship, but the swimming pool was filled direct from the Nile River.)

Animals. Don't sleep with your pets or allow them to lick your face, since they may harbor worms and parasites. Observe pets carefully. If they act lethargic or ill without obvious cause, have distended stomachs (hanging low), or you see ricelike worms around their rectum or in feces, have them dewormed. Keep their quarters clean. Do not let them eat off your plates. Teach your children to wash their hands *with soap* immediately after petting or touching any animal. Even if you do not own a cat, cover backyard sandboxes and wear gloves when gardening, because stray animals use flower beds and other soft soils as a litter box. Do not walk barefoot through barnyards or rain puddles that might be contaminated by animal feces, especially when traveling.

———

To test for parasites, a doctor will provide a kit containing instructions and materials to collect a stool sample for laboratory analysis. Tests are not always accurate, but once a parasite has been identified, naturopathic, Chinese, and Ayurvedic doctors are highly experienced in using safe natural substances for elimination. Many herbs prevent and cure parasites, but don't try to deal with them on your own. Parasites are notoriously difficult to eliminate. Doctors trained in alternative medicine typically focus on boosting the overall immune system to restore the body's natural defense mechanisms and balance. Refer to the Anti-Protozoa Program in appendix C for information and discuss it with your doctor.

PART II

The Most Effective Nondrug Therapies

CHAPTER 9

Neurofeedback: Retraining Brain Waves

Explaining her addictions, Nicole says, "I always felt 'off,' like something wasn't quite right in my brain, so I had to fix myself, not knowing, of course, what it was I was fixing." The trauma of her father's death when she was twelve spurred her use of recreational drugs for a quick fix to ease her emotional pain. Only thirty years later did she learn that both her father's brother and a cousin had committed suicide as a result of deep depression, and that her problem was rampant in the family tree.

"It was the early 1970s. I was about sixteen, living in West Hollywood, and using drugs, alcohol, or cigarettes was extremely easy. Everybody you looked up to had drugs. That was just what you did." At first, smoking pot was recreational, but her use escalated and "got out of hand," so Nicole quit briefly.

After high school, she decided to learn through travel, going to Israel, where she lived for a year, then to Germany, around Europe, and throughout Canada. Wherever she went, "I was using drugs right and left." There was never a problem finding a source. "It's like an animal instinct. You meet up with people and you just *know*. Back then, it was pretty loose, not like it is now."

Returning home, Nicole got married in 1977, and soon had two boys. During both pregnancies and nursing, she didn't smoke and stopped using drugs and alcohol. "I quit because I was really into nursing and interested in babies," she says. "Nursing helps take care of something in your brain, but as soon as I stopped, I went back on drugs."

"When I wasn't taking drugs, I didn't feel normal. I felt anxious or depressed. It would go back and forth. When I was on something, I was able to focus, work, and live—until it wasn't okay."

By the mid-1980s, Nicole's drug use had escalated again and the family urged her to join Narcotics Anonymous. She attended for six years, staying clear of street drugs until the early 1990s, when she suffered a breakdown accompanied by deep depression.

Doctors put her on Prozac and other antidepressants, but Nicole is a noncompliant patient. "I never listened to doctors. I knew how to self-medicate. If they told me to take one, I would take two. If they said take two, I would take one. As soon as I felt better, I stopped because I didn't think I needed them."

Her mother's decline into Alzheimer's deepened Nicole's depression until she rarely got out of bed except to visit her mother or drive her son, an actor, to auditions. "My kids just had to fend for themselves. One Christmas I barely got out of bed to watch them open gifts, and then I started crying and went back to sleep," she recalls. "But you can't sleep for twenty-four hours, so when I woke up I would take Vicodin with beer to put me back to sleep. I did not want to be conscious. I wanted to be *gone*."

Referred to a new therapist who did blood tests, a written test, and talked to her at length, Nicole was asked, "Do you have episodes of mania?" "I wasn't quite sure what he was talking about, and then I said, 'Oh yeah. I've always been an extremist—totally up or totally down, never a happy medium, ever.'"

Finally diagnosed as bipolar, Nicole was already thirty pounds overweight before lithium therapy added close to fifty pounds in two months. "You're not supposed to take lithium if you have thyroid problems, which I do, plus I was allergic to it. But they gave it to me anyway, never fully explaining all the side effects of lithium. I realized, this is so not right and I felt I was so out of touch with reality, totally in my own little world, which wasn't a good place to be in."

The next two years Nicole calls "the dead years," when she mostly stayed in bed, becoming even more depressed, obese, and isolated.

A close friend needed a ride to a local biofeedback clinic, so Nicole drove her. While waiting for her friend, she read literature on using neurofeedback to correct brain-wave imbalances associated with depression, bipolar disorder, anxiety, autism, addictions, sleep disorders, Tourette's syndrome, seizures, chronic pain, and autoimmune disorders.

Nicole signed up for treatment with Dr. Victoria L. Ibric, M.D., Ph.D., B.C.I.A.C., D.A.B.P.S.[1] A former Romanian oncologist with thirty years' experience in cancer research, therapy, and neurology, Dr. Ibric has for the last twelve years taught neurofeedback and biofeedback while maintaining a private biofeedback clinic in Pasadena, California. Nicole felt she had "nothing else to do and nothing to lose."

Sensors attached to a person's scalp with a dab of conductive paste are connected to an electroencephalogram (EEG) that displays on a computer the different brain waves occurring. Nicole put on glasses with red, blue, or white lenses. "Your eyes are closed, but you see flashing lights, which do something to the brain. Your mind trails into different directions. Half the time I fell asleep, but it worked even then."

Nicole was being treated with a type of neurofeedback called the ROSHI technique. Unlike conventional neurofeedback, ROSHI presents the brain with a series of flashing lights that are intended to dislodge "stuck" brain-wave patterns. Among neurofeedback practitioners, it is considered somewhat experimental, although very effective with some patients.

Uncharacteristically persistent, Nicole attended forty-five-to-sixty-minute sessions three times a week for eight months, then once or twice a week, then every other week. "Why I kept going, when it took so long, I have no idea. I just knew this was something: a light at the end of the tunnel after so many years of darkness."

After six weeks, Nicole spontaneously stopped smoking and reduced her alcohol consumption. "I didn't even want to quit smoking; I just realized I had. I haven't smoked now in seven years." After a couple of months, she weaned herself off lithium and Prozac. "Doctors told me I would be on some type of medication for the rest of my life, and I thought, 'I am *not*—I don't like how it's making me feel.'" She also began to walk every morning at 6 A.M., joined a gym, worked out daily, and lost weight.

When Dr. Ibric started Nicole on a new treatment protocol designed to improve interhemispheric synchronization, Nicole's level of energy increased and stayed high for a full week. Her progress from these weekly sessions was described by the doctor as "remarkable." She no longer used any pharmaceutical or recreational drugs, alcohol, or cigarettes and had no depression.

Today, when Nicole begins to feel any anxiety or depression returning, she stops by Dr. Ibric's clinic on her way to work for a single neurofeedback session that rebalances her brain waves and lasts several months.

Already taking certain amino acids as part of her therapy with Dr. Ibric, Nicole read Julia Ross's books *The Diet Cure* and *The Mood Cure*[2] and made an appointment with this successful substance-abuse counselor at her clinic, Recovery Systems.[3] Along with daily vitamins, minerals, and fish oils, Nicole began taking more amino acids: two tyrosine three times a day; two phenylalanine a couple times a day; and 5-HTP in the late afternoon. "The aminos just put everything up a notch," she explains.

"Neurofeedback quite simply saved my life," she says. "Life is great now. I've been married twenty-five years. I have my kids and a new grandson. Funnily enough, I work in a rehab hospital for drug, alcohol, and chronic depression, with patients exactly like me."

Retraining Brain Waves

Brain cells (neurons) transmit messages in the form of electrical impulses from one cell to another. The brain's signaling functions, processing of sensory information, programming of motor and emotional responses, learning, and memory are carried out by interconnected sets of neurons. There are about 50 billion neurons in the cortex, each of which has about 100,000 connections with other neurons. This network of neurons and their interconnections generate electrical signals that can be measured at the scalp. These trillions of electrical impulses take on rhythmic patterns, or "waves," that spread across large areas of the brain's surface and can be recorded on electroencephalograms (EEGs).

Neurofeedback was discovered in the 1960s by several groups of researchers. The father of contemporary neurofeedback is Professor Emeritus Barry Sterman of the University of California Los Angeles School of Medicine. He discovered that laboratory cats, when trained through operant conditioning to increase a certain range of brain waves (SMR [sensorimotor rhythm] or 12–15 Hz), had greatly increased resistance to developing seizure activity after exposure to toxic chemicals that usually produced seizures.

The first work that Sterman did with humans was to help patients with chronic seizures and poor medication responses become seizure-free. Sterman and his students went on to develop these techniques into more refined approaches to brain biofeedback, which included the treatment of ADHD, brain injuries, anxiety, depression and other mental disorders associated with EEG dysfunction in the brain.[4]

Biofeedback, the science from which neurofeedback evolved, has been very successful in teaching patients to consciously regulate automatic body functions, such as heart rate and blood pressure, and to reeducate damaged muscles. Using computer technology with a feedback loop, a patient is taught how to mentally ask his body to do something specific, like lower his blood pressure. The computer monitors the blood pressure and turns on a light or creates a sound when it dips, allowing the patient to learn through repetition how to lower it at will, without computer assistance.

By 2000, biofeedback was such a success that about half of major insurance companies covered the therapy for some forty conditions, including chronic pain, high blood pressure, migraine headaches, and ADD.[5] The fastest-growing area of biofeedback became neurofeedback (*neuro* referring to the nervous system), using EEGs to measure brain-wave activity and enable patients to deliberately change it.

Traditional neurofeedback is very straightforward. A patient sits in front of a computer screen and is connected to a very small EEG recorder with thin wires and electrodes that are pasted to the scalp. The therapist uses the computer readings to assess the proper or improper level of brain waves at any frequency and then sets up a program that rewards desirable frequencies and inhibits damaging frequencies with sounds and computer visualizations.[6]

There are several types of brain waves recorded, but five are most often examined: beta, SMR (sensorimotor rhythm), alpha, theta, and delta. Each has a distinct *frequency*, measured in cycles per second (or hertz), and *amplitude* (range of oscillation), measured in millionths of a volt. Different frequencies and amplitudes correspond to various states of arousal and activities.[7]

Beta waves (15–18 Hz) occur when we are fully awake, with eyes open, and concentrating on something. They are also stimulated when we study anything novel but disappear during repetitive problem solving. Considered a measure of arousal, higher frequencies of beta (21–30 Hz), not a desirable frequency, can indicate anxiety and obsessions. Traditional neurofeedback often rewards beta-wave activity in order to increase brain activity, to relieve depression, or to improve concentration in individuals with ADHD.

SMR waves (12–15 Hz) are associated with calm attention and with physical inactivity. A cat generates huge amounts of SMR brain waves when it is waiting motionless for its prey to get close. A hyperactive child learns to calm down through neurofeedback that rewards and increases the ability to generate SMR waves. Generally, disturbances in

SMR are not associated with depression or mania, although SMR training can be very calming to someone in an agitated or manic state.[8]

Alpha waves (8–12 Hz), when recorded with our eyes closed, are an indicator of relaxed wakefulness and meditative states. People emitting excessive alpha frequency, however, may either be quite "spacey" or anxious. Higher alpha activity is associated with creativity, one's ability to originate new ideas, but not with intelligence—the capacity to learn and understand. Stimulation that comes when the eyes are open decreases alpha waves, as does a state of danger or high alert. Brain waves change with age, and the alpha frequency diminishes in children as they mature.[9] In general, alpha frequency is gradually reduced as we age. Neurofeedback can often raise this, increasing mental acuity and the rate and quality of thinking in older persons.

Excessive alpha activity on the left side of the brain may be associated with depression. Treatment protocols that reduce left frontal alpha-wave activity while increasing left frontal beta-wave activity (15–18 Hz) are quite effective in treating depression.[10]

Theta waves (4–7 Hz) are associated with light, healthy sleep. Although the normal adult produces no theta rhythm while awake, these frequencies are important in infancy, childhood, and young adults, and they indicate pleasure. Children with concentration problems are often found to have excessive theta activity in the front of their brains, where mental processing takes place. So while they are awake in class trying to concentrate, their brain is literally half-asleep. Neurofeedback corrects this by teaching the child how to reduce theta waves. Theta disturbances are not usually associated with mood problems, but with problems of attention and self-regulation.[11]

Delta waves (0.5–3 Hz) are found mostly during periods of deep sleep, but do appear in small amounts during the day in both men and women, increasing around noon and peaking around 4 P.M.[12]

In a 2002 *Psychiatric Times* interview of Siegfried Othmer, Ph.D., chief scientist at EEG Spectrum International, Inc.,[13] neurofeedback was recommended as an "adjunctive" or additional treatment for the psychiatric disorders ADHD, anxiety, post-traumatic stress disorder, phobias, obsessive-compulsive and bipolar disorders, and depression, as well as autism and addictive disorders.[14] Other sources indicate that it is helpful in addressing Tourette's syndrome, seizures, sleep disorders, substance abuse, and chronic fatigue.[15]

The science underlying neurofeedback is exceedingly complex. According to Henry Mann, M.D., a psychiatrist and neurofeedback therapist, "Neurofeedback today is often preceded with the administration of a quantitative EEG or brain map that measures brain activity and compares it to a database of 'normal' people. This 'map' is used to guide treatment. A common finding on brain maps of depressed persons is excessive communication and linking of the alpha waves between the left and right prefrontal cortex, which is just above the eyes, that can be treated with neurofeedback.

"In addition to the ROSHI treatment described earlier for Nicole, there are other novel treatments that are quite effective with depression, including the LENS (Low Energy Neurofeedback System) and hemoencephalography. LENS utilizes small amounts of electromagnetic energy to reduce 'blocked' brain waves at nineteen different sites on the scalp. This unlocking allows the brain to begin to function at optimal capacity. Its inventor, Len Ochs, describes the process as 'taking the logs off a railroad track.'[16]

"Hemoencephalography (HEG) involves training the brain to increase blood flow, usually to the regions of the brain directly behind the forehead, which is where the executive functions and control systems of the brain are located. This is the area of the brain that distinguishes people from other mammals and is the center of thought, planning, self-regulation and emotional self-control. HEG teaches us to exercise this part of our brains and increase its strength in much the same way that physical exercise increases stamina and cardiac strength. HEG treatment is helpful with ADHD, bipolar disorder and depression, as well as other brain function disorders."[17]

Neurofeedback takes between twenty and forty sessions, and appears to be effective regardless of whether a disorder is due to unknown causes, childhood or subsequent trauma, or genetic tendencies. (The

LENS treatment may take about half that length of time.) The best way to locate a practitioner near you is through the International Society for Neuronal Regulation's provider system (www.isnr.org).

D. Corydon Hammond, Ph.D., professor and psychologist at the University of Utah School of Medicine, says neuroscientists have discovered a brain-wave pattern that identifies people with a "biological predisposition for developing depression." In the left frontal area of the brain, there is an excess of slow, alpha brain-wave activity that indicates a vulnerability to depression. According to Dr. Hammond, research has found that antidepressants have only an 18 percent effect over and above the placebo effects, and medications appear "to still leave intact the biological predisposition for becoming more easily depressed."[18] By retraining the brain, it is possible to produce an enduring change that does not require taking medication indefinitely.

CHAPTER 10

Releasing Trauma by Eye Movement Desensitization & Reprocessing or Emotional Transformation Therapy

Gina grew up in Colorado in a seemingly idyllic two-parent family. Her father was a teacher who worked extra jobs to support the family. They were athletic, "enjoying skiing, tennis, and everything very active," says Gina.

Home was not paradise, in spite of external appearances. Gina's father was absent most of the time, working and drinking. "From elementary school on, I had to be a people pleaser, wanted to do everything perfect so I wasn't the cause of my dad's occasional drinking rages and fights with mom.

"As early as I can remember, I survived on about four hours of sleep a night. In school, I was a straight-A student, but it was difficult for me. I had a hard time remembering things, sorting out my thoughts, and staying organized. My friends could study for a test once. I always had major anxiety before even the simplest tests and would take notes, study, and restudy." An overachiever, Gina also had a part-time job to pay for horseback riding and to save for college.

Always being busy, not sleeping, and working too much finally caught up with her. A sore throat and no energy were first diagnosed as a throat infection, treated with antibiotics. When symptoms continued, a chiropractor diagnosed mononucleosis. "I slept for about six weeks and was on vitamins. My body went from that of a competitive athlete to not being able to do anything," she says.

Severe seasonal allergies, having wisdom teeth pulled, and a collapsed lung during high school made maintaining the "perfect child" role increasingly difficult. "I was happy on the outside, but on the inside I was an emotional wreck," says Gina. "I did not share my feelings with anyone, including myself. The true emotions were buried deep inside."

During her first semester of college, Gina received a low grade in physiology. "It was my first C ever. I was devastated and had a breakdown. That's when I started seeing psychologists, trying to understand how my past affected me, why I have to be perfect."

In spite of the meltdown, Gina later graduated from college with honors. Afterward, "I married my high school sweetheart, the love of my life," she says. "He was a wonderful husband—also a workaholic perfectionist who shared my work ethic and need to please."

Gina began a teaching career, becoming obsessed, spending endless hours on the job. "I couldn't just teach from eight to three. I had to do all the extra programs that needed to be done and no one else wanted to do.

"My husband's profession took us on a journey to making more money than we ever dreamed of and moving away from family and friends in order to climb the corporate ladder to success." With each move, his career and network of business friends grew stronger, but as a teacher, Gina had to reapply and start all over in each new district. At each location, she took on more responsibility and struggled to work with peers who often didn't want to match her efforts.

Anxiety attacks over work and uncontrollable crying during the night or after being intimate with her husband prompted more trips to the psychologist. "On the outside, I maintained the happy, joyful, self-confident image, but on the inside I was beating myself up and had little confidence, although I was receiving teaching awards and praise from my peers. I was getting through the day but emotionally just shutting down."

A California therapist used relaxation and hypnosis to help reduce Gina's anxiety, but, Gina admits, "I was never honest with her in terms of the other deeper intimacy issues that I could not deal with." Gina found a new practitioner to address her low self-esteem. She also changed jobs, joining a "wonderful" principal and staff who shared her passion to reach "hard to teach" children. "I began to seek a balance between work and taking care of myself," she recalls.

By the next move, to Washington State, Gina's husband was earning enough that she no longer had to work. "I thought, dream of all dreams—to be a stay-at-home wife, living a life of luxury. He went on as usual, and I started feeling for the first time like I had no purpose in life."

Gina fell into depression. Loving and supportive as always, her husband suggested that she take up riding horses again at a nearby stable and find a part-time job to keep busy, since he was still constantly traversing the globe on business. "I went from compulsive workaholism into an addiction to horses," says Gina. "For two years, I was at the barn seven days a week."

When a friend told her about a part-time position at a Christian preschool, Gina decided to return to teaching, but after a few months found herself even more depressed and lethargic. "I began lying to my husband. He'd come home and wonder why the laundry wasn't done or things like that, and I would make up stories. I'd really just come home from work and sleep."

A friend suggested that the perpetually gray, rainy weather might be causing seasonal affective disorder (SAD). After a quick interview, Gina's general practitioner put her on Prozac. "Although the depression lifted a little, I began having difficulty sleeping. My husband was on another extended business trip. When he called each night, he noticed that my speech was more and more rapid and I was having difficulty staying focused, even in short conversations. I told him I was not sleeping very well." The truth was she was not sleeping at all. After seven days, she went to see the doctor again. Feeling that her mania might be a reaction to Prozac, he prescribed sleeping pills to accompany the drug.

Gina turned on her car radio after leaving the doctor's office, hearing news of the Columbine High School shooting in Colorado. "This tragedy sent me over the edge and I began having hallucinations about rescuing children. My husband returned from his trip to find me talking nonstop, planning grandiose world-saving missions." The next day, Gina prepared to go teach dressed in *Sleepless in Seattle* pajamas and a Denver Broncos baseball hat, carrying a box stuffed with favorite childhood things for "show and tell." Her husband called the doctor, who sent them to the hospital.

Admitted to the psychiatric ward, Gina was diagnosed as bipolar and put on Depakote, Klonopin, Ativan, and Zyprexa, but nothing seemed to help. A new doctor in the rotation switched her to lithium and sleep medications. "After a ten-day visit to the psych ward, I was sent home to begin my life on a cocktail of drugs and biweekly doctor visits. I really don't remember much except sleeping twelve to fourteen hours a day, living this completely hazed, dazed life, going to psychiatrists and psychologists. I was trying to get to the root of my problem while under the influence of drugs," Gina recalls. "But I could never find the root of anything, because I couldn't think or remember from one day to the next. I carried a notepad around with me because I forgot everything. And I gained thirty pounds from the lithium."

After three months on several psychiatric drugs, however, Gina was functioning better and "I felt like I was finally seeing the light at the end of a very dark tunnel." A trip to Europe with her parents was a welcome escape. During the trip, old family issues and emotions began to surface, but once home, before she could probe these feelings, Gina crashed into severe depression again. "I began having suicidal thoughts and withdrawing from everything around me," she says.

Her husband said he wanted a divorce a few weeks later. The news triggered cycles of all-day depression and all-night mania. Gina protested to the doctors, the lawyers, and her husband that the divorce should not be allowed to go through because she was sick. Under the law, however, it took only ninety days once the papers were served.

The night her divorce was final, while on the plane to Colorado to be close to family and friends, Gina realized that "I need to figure out on my own what is going on. I need to look for a doctor, somebody who is open to the pharmaceuticals but who will also listen if I find something else and be willing to try it."

Gina found such a doctor in Denver to help her manage the medications, cope with the loss of her marriage, and address old issues. "I said, 'I can't live like this. I've been in therapy before and there was always something that I didn't exactly understand. Nothing seems to help.'" After a few sessions, the therapist recommended Eye Movement Desensitization & Reprocessing (EMDR, explained later), saying it could accomplish in three months what might take three times as long using conventional therapy.

"I had no understanding of what EMDR was or how tapping on my knees or holding on to vibrating paddles was going to help me," recalls Gina. "The technique helped me deal with intimacy issues I had never addressed with my husband. By going through EMDR, I finally got to the root of my anxieties, which was sexual abuse."

When Gina was an adolescent, she had suffered two separate incidents of sexual fondling—by a neighborhood boy and by an older cousin. These had colored her perspective on intimacy, affecting all her relationships. "My dad would sometimes have bouts of rage after drinking binges, and I was afraid if I told my mother [about the sexual abuse], she would tell my father, and if he ever found out, he would kill them. I knew this boy and my cousin weren't supposed to be doing what they were doing, and the anxiety just kept coming back. I was with my husband for twenty-two years, but intimacy issues were always there. In the middle of being intimate with him, I'd have anxiety attacks."

After the divorce, Gina rented an apartment in the back of the house where she grew up. "Before the therapy, I'd be in the backyard mowing the lawn, and I'd get close to the back fence, or look out the window and see a person in the backyard, and get these anxious feelings." EMDR changed all that within three months. "In the sessions, I'd go to the anxiety and, using visualization techniques, try to identify the scene. It kept coming back to this house I grew up in." From the visual image, Gina realized that a close childhood friend was present as well.

She telephoned him, saying, "'I just keep having a vision of this man doing something to me. Do you remember anything?' He said, 'Yes, and he molested me too.'" The friend had never told anyone either. For years, the young man had been suppressing his guilt with cocaine, marijuana, and alcohol. When Gina called him about the incident, he was in recovery. The friend confided that he had been unable to kick the addictions until he had addressed this long-ago sexual abuse.

Says Gina, "I was kind of carrying a monkey on my back, and after EMDR, it was suddenly gone. I was finally able to talk to my dad and mom about it."

Gina remained on lithium during EMDR therapy, but feeling dramatically improved and hating the drug side effects, she investigated natural vitamin treatments to replace the drug. Discovering Equilib™,[1] an all-natural vitamin/mineral/amino acid supplement specifically formulated for people with emotional disorders, she began taking the supplement and gradually weaned herself off lithium. Within two months, all Gina's bipolar symptoms were gone.

When she was first diagnosed, Gina was told she would be on lithium or some other prescription mood stabilizer for the rest of her life, and she would probably never be able to work full time again. Today, she uses only Equilib™ and maintains a very strict diet, controlling her intake of refined sugars and carbohydrates. She has not needed a psychiatrist since completing EMDR and beginning the supplement and nutrition program.

Gina began volunteering at a residential day treatment facility when she first returned to Denver, working with students suffering from mental health disorders. After her recovery, she became an employee at the facility and is working to educate her peers about alternative treatments for bipolar disorder. She is also completing a master's degree in special education, seeking an opportunity to assist emotionally disturbed children through alternative treatments and a nutritionally oriented program.

Eye Movement Desensitization & Reprocessing (EMDR)

Alcoholism is prevalent in Gina's family, suggesting that genetics may play a role in her bipolar disorder. The Equilib™ vitamin/mineral/ amino acid supplements probably would have ended her mood swings, as they have for thousands of people, but supplements alone might not have uprooted the emotional trauma entrenched in Gina's subconscious as a result of the childhood sexual molestation.

Traumatic experiences, such as rape, sexual or physical abuse, having an abortion, war experiences, being the victim of a violent crime, or terrifying accidents often cause post-traumatic stress disorder (PTSD). The incident overwhelms a person's normal defense mechanisms and results in intense fear, feelings of being trapped and helplessness, or of losing control, often accompanied by tremendous guilt, for an act or for having survived in situations where others died. Symptoms of PTSD may include depression, anxiety attacks, rage or aggressive behavior, suicidal tendencies, substance abuse, terrifying nightmares, and visual flashbacks in which the person reexperiences some of the emotions and sensations from the original trauma.

According to the EMDR Institute in California, eye movement desensitization and reprocessing has rapidly risen to prominence in treating both acute and chronic PTSD because of its speed and effectiveness in releasing these memories. EMDR is now given the same status as cognitive therapy in the American Psychiatric Association's 2004 *Practice Guideline for the Patients with Acute Stress Disorder and Posttraumatic Stress Disorder*. EMDR is one of three methods recommended for treatment of victims of terrorism in the Israeli National Council for Mental Health 2002 Guidelines, and one of four therapies given the highest level of evidence and recommendation in the U.S. Department of Veterans Affairs and the U.S. Department of Defense 2004 Clinical Practice Guidelines for PTSD.[2]

Women may experience abortion as a traumatic event, especially if they are forced into an unwanted procedure by husbands, boyfriends, parents, or others. If the woman has been the victim of sexual assault or domestic abuse, a coerced decision may be perceived as the ultimate violation, leading to higher rates of depression, mood disorders, self-harm, and suicide.[3]

EMDR was developed by Francine Shapiro, Ph.D., senior research fellow at the Mental Research Institute in Palo Alto, California, after she noticed her own stress reactions diminish when her eyes swept back and forth as she walked through a park. The therapy is used around the world to "reprogram" the brains of trauma victims and release them from the psychic pain of continually reliving elements of their experience.

The cerebrum, our largest brain mass, has two halves: gray matter that originates and processes nerve impulses, and white matter that transmits those impulses. Its cerebral cortex (what we visualize as our brain) has a beige covering tucked and folded into hundreds of grooves and fissures.[4] This neocortex, or "new bark," is linked to every part of the body. Here, cognitive thinking that set humans apart takes place— perception, attention, impulse inhibition, language, learning, planning, and conscience.[5]

The limbic system, one of the first parts of the brain to evolve, rests atop the brain stem roughly in the center of the head. This is mood headquarters, the source of emotions and instinctive reactions, with survival being its highest priority. Danger is handled by a committee— the hippocampus, amygdala, hypothalamus, pituitary, and thalamus.

The hippocampus stores short-term memories and a few long-term memories, but sends most of the latter to the cerebral cortex for safekeeping. The amygdala processes all emotional information and works with the hippocampus and neocortex to decide on the appropriate emotional response. Is there really a snake in the grass or is it just a mistaken stick? Only then does the hypothalamus (with the amygdala) tell the body how to respond, sending messages to our pea-sized pituitary gland, which directs production of all hormones, for a rush shipment of adrenaline. The thalamus is a relay station for all incoming sensory messages (except smell), sending them on to appropriate brain centers.[6]

Because the emotional brain is an earlier, more rudimentary structure, it is faster than the thinking brain. When we are very frightened, the limbic system can take over, superseding rational brain activity, focusing all resources on survival in that moment, which is why we may become "irrational" under stress.

Any experience with a high emotional impact is preserved in long-term memory as a survival mechanism to assist in perceiving and handling future threats. These memories may surface, again and again, after the event is past, however, causing PTSD, a perpetual reliving of the stored-up feelings and sensations. Sometimes, when the incident occurred very early in life or is based on a series of similar, repetitive events spread years apart, the event may not even be consciously remembered and remain out of reach in the subconscious.

The primary objective of treatment is to "reprogram" the emotional brain so it stops continuing to react based on past experiences. EMDR and Emotional Transformation Therapy™ (ETT) (discussed later) are exceptionally effective because they use methods that access the emotional brain via the body, rather than through rational talk therapy, quickly accessing deeply buried feelings and responses.

What does EMDR therapy involve? The institute's informative Web site, www.emdr.com (which has a link to a list of trained clinicians), describes eight phases of treatment.

In Phase 1, the therapist takes a patient's history, assesses whether EMDR would be appropriate and the patient's "readiness," and develops a plan. In Phase 2, the therapist ensures that a patient is relatively stable and has good coping skills and methods for dealing with emotional distress. In Phases 3 through 6, the patients identify the most vivid visual image related to the incident, or negative belief about themselves, along with the emotions and body sensations related to the incident or belief.

Patients are then taught to focus on the image, negative thoughts, or sensations, while simultaneously moving their eyes back and forth, following the therapist's fingers across their field of vision, for twenty to thirty seconds. Although eye movements are most commonly used, auditory tones, tapping on the body, or other methods may be used to create a stimulus that requires a kind of dual attention.

Next, patients are told to "let their mind go," observing whatever thought, feeling, image, memory, or sensation that comes to the surface. The therapy involves helping them "process the association" before moving on to the next focus. If images cause distress, the practitioner uses procedures that both ease the condition and aid in the processing.

Phase 7 is closure, in which the patient is asked to keep a journal of issues that may arise. Phase 8 is a reevaluation of the patient's progress. Throughout, the overall goal is to produce the most comprehensive treatment in the shortest period of time for patients, while maintaining their emotional stability.

Numerous clinical studies have demonstrated EMDR's efficiency. In 2002, *The Journal of Clinical Psychology* reported that both EMDR and prolonged exposure therapy produced a significant reduction in PTSD and depression symptoms, finding that 70 percent of EMDR participants achieved an outcome in three active treatment sessions, compared to 29 percent of those in prolonged talk therapy, and EMDR had fewer dropouts.[7] A 1998 meta-analysis of studies determined that EMDR and behavior therapy were superior to psychopharmaceuticals and that EMDR was more efficient than behavior therapy, with results obtained in one-third the time.[8]

Emotional Transformation Therapy™

A new form of visual light stimulation, Emotional Transformation Therapy (ETT™), is emerging that quickly relieves a wide range of mood disorders. The use of light therapy began in 1982, when D. F. Kripke demonstrated that artificial light could alter mood states and N. E. Rosenthal reported the antidepressant effect of light exposure on a bipolar patient.[9] Since then, exposure to artificial white light has become a conventionally accepted treatment for seasonal affective disorder (SAD).

SAD is a type of depression estimated to affect between 3 and 5 percent of the population, occurring primarily in winter or at latitudes when daylight is shortened. It is also seen in shift workers and geriatric patients confined indoors with little natural light or as a result of jet lag, conditions that disrupt the body's internal clock, the circadian rhythm.[10] Treatment simply involves seating patients in front of special full-spectrum, bright white lights of 10,000 lux for thirty to sixty minutes, usually each morning during the light-deprived period, to lift depression and reduce excessive sleeping, carbohydrate cravings, and lethargy. Research in the 1990s showed that such light exposure consistently increased blood serotonin levels in both depressed patients and healthy controls.[11] White light therapy, however, works for only 47 percent of SAD patients and must be used daily because it does not eradicate the problem, but simply alleviates symptoms.[12]

Emotional Transformation Therapy™ is an accelerated form of psychotherapy that combines the use of colored lights, eye movement and stimulation, and brain-wave entrainment with psychotherapy processes to eradicate emotional problems. Developed by Steven Vazquez, Ph.D., a practicing therapist for twenty-five years, ETT™ provides rapid, in-depth relief of depression, post-traumatic stress disorder, anxiety disorders, and physical pain.

People often connect moods with colors, saying they feel *blue* or dislike *gray* overcast days because they are so depressing. ETT™ uses a small light instrument to project beams of low-brightness light of different colors into the patient's eyes while the verbal processing of emotional issues takes place under a trained practitioner's guidance.

In 1977, Harvard psychiatrist Frederick Schiffer found that the left portions of both eyes access the brain's right hemisphere while the right portions of both eyes access the left hemisphere, introducing the ability to elicit emotions through the eyes. EMDR uses roughly three basic angles for eye movement to aid elimination of unconscious issues. ETT™ utilizes eye positions in twenty-four different angles through a 360-degree range of peripheral eye positions. According to Dr. Vazquez, this brings forth previously fixed, unconscious, emotional states and allows them to be transformed within minutes.

In 1939 it was discovered that pulsating light into the eyes causes brain-wave patterns to align with the light's pulse, one of the processes utilized in neurofeedback. By 1991, Michael Hutchison described several devices that use light stimulation to entrain brain waves.[13] ETT™ takes this approach a step further, using the knowledge that helpful insights, emotions, or relevant memories are more easily retrieved during brain-wave patterns of eight to eleven cycles per second and combines light therapy with psychotherapy techniques.

Accessing memories, emotions, or sensations deep in the unconscious mind is one of the major challenges of psychotherapy. Hypnosis is sometimes used for this, but many people are not hypnotizable. Others are highly susceptible to suggestion during hypnotic states, risking the creation of false memories. Body-oriented therapies like craniosacral manipulation or trigger-point massage therapies can release unconscious memories, but often without the aid of a psychotherapist to help the patient understand what occurred. Since touch is not acceptable in most psychotherapy, ETT™ uses rhythmic-colored lights along with eye movement and stimulation to reach deeply buried, unconscious emotions. When combined with psychotherapy, the emerging emotional states can be rapidly and consistently transformed, stopping the unwanted emotions and providing understanding.

Preliminary studies have demonstrated significant reduction in SAD symptoms from ETT™,[14] and cases reported in two articles in *Annals*, the journal of the American Psychotherapy Association, in 2004 and 2005 demonstrate its speed and effectiveness for SAD and PTSD.[15, 16] Although based on well-tested therapies, ETT™ is relatively new, so except for the above references, little about it has been published to date. For more information, go to www.lightworkassociates.com.

CHAPTER 11

Reconnecting Mind and Body: Prayer, Affirmations, Imagery, Yoga, and Meditation

Andrea Schmook's first diagnosis was acute paranoid schizophrenia, then schizo-affective disorder, and, finally, manic-depression. She chuckles remembering her initial episode in 1977. Believing she was the Virgin Mary, Andrea donned her husband's blue jeans, put her best long green-and-white polka-dot dress on top, and veiled her head with the cover from the birds' cage. Leading her two children, their neighborhood friends, a dog on a leash in one hand, caged birds in the other, she formed a procession that arrived at the children's school around ten o'clock one morning. State police rapidly converged, delivering Andrea to the Alaska Psychiatric Institute, where, within ten minutes, she was admitted and drugged against her will with Haldol.

It was a nightmare experience, says Andrea. "The Haldol increased all the hallucinations, delusions, and voices. It didn't take anything away—it made things worse. Plus, it shut my body down." All her muscles became rigid, making it hard to unbend her arms or move her legs. Her teeth were clenched together and wouldn't open. "I made up my mind I would *never* go back to a mental institution again."

The odds were against her. As she was being discharged, the nurse handed her a bag of medications, saying she must keep them with her at all times and never go off them. The nurse's parting observation was this: "You'll be in and out of here for the rest of your life because you're going back to the same situation that caused this." Andrea was determined to defy the odds. "I told myself, 'No I'm not. I'm not *ever* coming back here. I am going to get better, and when I get better, I'm going to help other people so they can do it too.'"

Her friends and family promised they would never take her to a mental hospital again, and, if she were picked up by the police and admitted again, they would get a court order for her release. They vowed to care for her at home whenever necessary.

After that, Andrea had two or three episodes a year that should have landed her in the hospital, each lasting around ten days. "My family would get together at one house and give me medications that just shut me down, put me to sleep," she says. They would rouse her sufficiently for spoon feedings and to take her to the bathroom. When an episode was over, they would tell her to get up, go home, go back to work, take care of her kids, and get on with life. "And that's what I would do," she says, "but the medication would leave me pretty drugged. I would be shaky. I could fall asleep at the drop of a hat, but I would go to work."

Even more remarkable than her family's support was the enlightened attitude at the engineering company where Andrea was employed as a secretary. Everyone knew about her illness, yet there was "absolutely no stigma or discrimination against me," she recalls. "When I'd get through an episode and go back, the engineers, surveyors, draftsmen, and other office workers would come in one by one and say, 'We're so happy you're back. You made it. You are going to get better and beat this thing. You're a survivor.'"

The whole mental health industry was a mystery to Andrea because it wasn't about regaining health. "Nobody ever got better! They tell you, you have to take this medication but you're never going to get better—your life is over. Why take the medication? It just didn't make any sense to me."

I said to myself, "I accept myself just the way I am, but what can I do about it?" Her sister gave Andrea a book that provided the answer—*Think and Grow Rich*. It asserted that whatever the mind can conceive and believe, it can achieve. As Andrea read, she learned about using affirmations. "Faith is built on changing belief systems inside your own conscious mind through affirmations. If you want to make changes, you write an affirmation, as if it has already happened," she says. "So I did."

Andrea wrote hundreds of different affirmations over the years and developed what she calls affirmative prayers. "We always pray like, 'Dear God, please give me a house, give me a job, give me a this or that,'" she explains. "As I studied scripture with mature, spiritual people, I discovered that you don't get what you want because you don't ask for the right things.

"What I needed to ask for was courage to get through this. Ask for the strength to work and earn a living so I could buy a house." It wasn't about praying for *things* but for internal attributes, "so that you become all that you were meant to be," which would ultimately bring the material possessions.

"I took my focus off what I didn't have because I had a mental illness," Andrea says, "and put my focus on what I did have—integrity and forgiveness and love and peace and personal power. I looked at all those things inside me, which was the Divine part of me. When I tapped into the Divine spirit—where the true power was—that combined my human and Divine spirit as one, and the healing began."

Andrea could sense when mania was approaching. "Before I had an episode, I always affirmed that 'the highest and best people are coming to me now. I *choose* to survive. I *have* beat this mental illness. I *am* recovered.'"

Often as part of a bipolar incident, rage would well up inside her against the emotional abuse her father had inflicted on the family. "I would take off in my car, drive down one-way streets the wrong way, because I couldn't figure out how to resolve this since my father was no longer living." Raised Russian Orthodox, she talked to the priest and tried confession, but neither helped.

One day as she drove around Anchorage in a crazed state, she wound up at the cemetery beside his grave. "I screamed at him. I yelled at him. I blamed him for my being mentally ill and for my life being so awful. When I got it all out, I knelt at his grave," she recalls. "I was able to say,

'And now I forgive you, because I realize you didn't do this on purpose. You thought you were doing this in my best interest. You did this out of love.'" Andrea felt so much better after releasing her anger that she was able to reduce her medications. Over time, she renamed the episodes. "These are healing crises, spiritual crises too, for the healing of that human spirit that was broken.

"I also learned, if you're trying to recover, you don't blame yourself, you don't blame others, you try to understand how the dynamics of relationships played in it, so that healing can happen."

Andrea was outraged when she emerged from one healing crisis to learn that her husband had called, saying that neither she nor their children could ever come home again. He wanted a divorce. A Vietnam veteran suffering from post-traumatic stress disorder (unknown and unnamed at that time), he was withdrawn, unable to give love, trapped in his own torments.

"I kept saying over and over, 'Why did he throw us out like we were garbage? Didn't he know we were the best thing he had?'" Her anger built. Finally her brother-in-law, Joe, who worked at the post office, sent the children and family members away, saying, "She's got to get this rage out." He had her lie down on the floor, surrounded and cushioned by pillows, then said, "What I want you to do, Andrea, is have a good old-fashioned temper tantrum. I want you to scream and yell, kick your feet, and I want you to cry, to get all of this out." She did, for several hours. "When I'd go through rage like this, it took a tremendous amount of energy, so what I would do afterwards was sleep. When I woke up from that session, oh boy, was there massive healing."

Although slowly getting better, Andrea was still on psychiatric drugs but found she needed fewer and lower doses following each healing crisis. One drug, Navane, may have triggered neuroleptic malignant syndrome, a rare but often fatal reaction. "I wound up in the hospital for six days with a fever of 106 degrees. I should never have been put on neuroleptics. They tell you you'll have dry mouth, blurred vision, stuff like that, but those real tough side effects—that can cause death—you never hear about.

"I made up my mind all along that I was going to be medication free." She continued using affirmations. Looking at the pill, "I would say out loud, 'I am now completely and totally free of all medications.' I would say that twenty times before I put it in my mouth."

On July 13, 1984, Andrea became manic, took money from her savings, and left Anchorage, driving blindly, without a plan. At Beaver Creek, in the Yukon Territory of Canada, the Royal Canadian Mounted Police picked her up and put her in jail in protective custody. She had no memory of who she was, where she had come from, or what had happened over the past few days. Finding her driver's license, they called her home, but there was no answer. So she was taken to a doctor's office to determine if she had been hurt or was on illegal drugs.

The doctor had another appointment, so he asked his nurse to come into the room and stay with Andrea. Coincidentally, just a year before, this Canadian nurse had become stranded in Anchorage because she ran out of money, and Andrea's sister had taken the woman in, given her a room, and helped her get a green card and a job, enabling her return to Canada. Only once during the nurse's stay did Andrea visit her sister's home for a few minutes, but the nurse now recognized Andrea immediately and telephoned the frantic family.

This was Andrea's last episode. She learned to recognize signs of oncoming mania. When a sensation began moving up her spine and her brain began to race, she would use relaxation and imagery techniques to halt the process.

"Years before, one Sunday morning in May, my husband and I were at Bishop Creek fishing," says Andrea. "He was down the creek and I was by myself when it started to rain. The smell of budding trees and flowers became stronger, fresh and clean. The raindrops hitting the water made little swirls and it was so incredibly peaceful."

Now whenever her mind would begin to race, she would go to a restroom or some other private place, and "I would close my eyes, start deep breathing, and tell myself, 'I am now relaxing completely and totally—breathe in, breathe out—totally relaxing,' I'd visualize myself back at Bishop Creek fishing, sensing all of the smells, sounds, and feelings again. It calmed me down and put me at peace in fifteen to twenty minutes," she recalls. "It didn't matter if people came in and out of the room, because I was totally unaware of them." Then Andrea would go back to whatever she had been doing when the symptoms began, doing mindless tasks for a while, gradually immersing herself in work that needed to get done that day but at a nonstressful pace to avoid slipping into mania.

Andrea also used creative imagery to move herself toward her ultimate goal: to be completely free of episodes and off medications. "I visualized the way I wanted my life to be and the way I wanted myself to be in the future. I wrote it out, and I would read it out loud to myself so I knew where I was going. It was really a vision of the future I wanted to live. There's tremendous power in a vision. If you don't know where you want to go, how will you know when you arrive?"

The "last piece of the puzzle" came when Andrea consulted a naturopathic physician, Dr. Cary Jasper. "He helped me a lot. I was still running on adrenaline all the time. He worked on my adrenal gland, gave me shots of natural stuff, and pills for the pancreas that helped calm me down.

"He told me to focus on eating complex carbohydrates. If I had meat, it should be no bigger than the palm of my hand, but to eat more rice, beans, fresh salads, and fresh veggies." He told her that anything to go into her mouth she should buy fresh from the produce section of the grocery store—no canned or frozen vegetables, nothing in a box. He explained that her constant anxiety, fear, and adrenaline intensity was because "you need more and more sugar all the time when you eat junk food. Complex carbohydrates give sugar your body needs—not a big jolt, just a little at a time, enough to carry you through the day without anxiety."

By learning to anticipate and stop the bipolar cycles, and by incorporating the lifestyle changes that Dr. Jasper taught her, Andrea soon no longer had any episodes and was able to stop taking all psychiatric drugs without any recurring symptoms.

The episode in 1984 was Andrea's last—more than twenty years ago. Uncertain when to declare herself totally recovered, she adopted the system used by cancer patients. After one year without an episode, "I really patted myself on the back." When she made it through the fifth year, "I knew this was *never* going to happen again. I beat it. I survived it. It is *gone!*"

Andrea considers herself very spiritual and wanted to give something back. She became a mental health advocate, working for the Governor's Advisory Council, helping create the first consumer organization for people with mental illness run by people *recovered* from mental illness. Called Mental Health Consumers of Alaska, it provides advocacy, peer support, and public education services, supporting those having any psychiatric diagnoses with care and finding jobs, housing, or food, much as her family had supported her.

Andrea worked as an outside contractor for the Elgin Mental Health Center in Chicago and later as the director of the Office of Consumer Affairs, charged with placing staff that had recovered from a mental disorder in all the hospitals. When requested to create a training program on recovery, Andrea took it a step further, developing what she called "A Vision of Recovery," first presented to the National Association of State Mental Health Program Directors. Splitting the attendees into two groups, she assigned one group to describe the state of mental health services today. "It was a sad picture of forced treatment, using the court system, people going into jails, losing their housing, living in poverty," she says. Andrea challenged the second group to "create a vision of what we would like tomorrow to be. The second group's vision included absolutely no stigma or discrimination against people with mental illness. People would be able to live wherever they chose. They would never lose their job," and so on. "It was like night and day."

Throughout the program, she emphasized how powerful visions are and explained how to train people to share your vision. Directors from all the other states were overwhelmed and thrilled.

Andrea's life has been irrevocably changed by her mental illness. "I'm not ashamed of it. I don't need to hide it. It really was a spiritual awakening and a transformation. You become a whole new person.

But when you're treated forcibly against your will, drugged with very powerful drugs, it stops the process. Many people get *stuck* right where they're at because nobody is helping them use this experience to transform their life."

To change the approach, Andrea started working on contract in 2003 through June 2005 for the state hospital in Anchorage where she was first admitted as a patient, setting up an Office of Consumer and Family Affairs. In July 2005, she was hired by the Anchorage Community Mental Health Center to be the director of consumer-directed services and was appointed by the governor to serve on the Alaska Mental Health Board.

She is board president of Peer Properties, a nonprofit organization that received a $250,000 state grant to establish a home for four women. "It's a beautiful house, with fireplaces, laundry facilities, and they each have a private entrance into their bedrooms."

Andrea says, "I've come full circle. I was raised in Alaska. I became mentally ill while I was a young adult and mother living in Alaska, received treatment at Alaska Psychiatric Institute and Anchorage Community Mental Health Services, and I recovered in Alaska. I left to see if my recovery would stick someplace else and it did. I returned to give back to my family and now work at the very two places where I had been treated. I've come home."

Affirmations

Andrea is not alone in perceiving her mental illness as a healing crisis that stimulated spiritual growth. Others interviewed for this book felt compelled to return to church during their healing journey or said in restrospect they were grateful for their illness because it utterly changed their lives in dramatic, positive ways.

Seldom does a person face death, or anything close to it, and emerge unchanged. In their darkest moment, many turn to a Divine entity, asking for assistance. Although healing does not necessarily follow immediately or sometimes ever, what often comes over time is an understanding of the ailment's higher purpose in stimulating a spiritual awakening. What comes is awareness of the guidance, received intuitively, about what steps to take next, and the amazing collection of "coincidences" that bring support during the process. What comes is the inner strength to somehow keep going toward your goal, even when you think you cannot.

In many religions, communication with the Divine is primarily through prayer. Another method is meditation, a conscious quieting of the mind's chatter that allows communion with the Universe or a Higher Self, our spirit or soul.

Affirmations and visualizations are also forms of inner communication used to change core beliefs and aid healing of depression, bipolar disorder, or other illnesses. Some people simply practice yoga for physical exercise. I have included it here because the centuries-old techniques were once primarily a spiritual practice used to open the chakras, energy channels (covered in the next chapter), that enhance the flow of life energy between body, mind, and spirit.

For twenty years one of the best-selling books on affirmations has been *You Can Heal Your Life* by Louise L. Hay.[1] Raped and abused as a child, Louise felt unloved and worthless, and spent her early adult life drawn to men who mistreated her. Gradually, through positive work experience, her self-esteem grew and she avoided abusive relationships because she no longer believed she deserved abuse. After a few years of menial jobs, she moved to New York, became a fashion model for big-name designers, and married into a world of international travel and wealth, but she still suffered from her early pattern of low self-esteem. When Louise's husband left her for another woman, she was devastated. Drawn to the Church of Religious Science in New York, she began "inner work," which led to becoming a transcendental meditator, took ministerial training, and eventually worked with others to heal physical illnesses by changing mental patterns.

Diagnosed with cancer, Louise was by then so confident of the mind/body connection that she felt that simply undergoing medical treatment to get rid of her cancer without clearing the mental patterns that created it would result in a recurrence. She investigated alternative ways of healing: using a therapist to release old bottled-up anger and resentment and finding a nutritionist to help cleanse and detoxify her body from all the junk foods she had eaten. All the while, she continued repeating positive affirmations for complete healing, heaping on herself the love and approval she had never received from others. After six months, Louise no longer needed treatment. Her cancer disappeared.

Louise believes, "Every thought we think is creating our future." Each chapter of her book begins with positive affirmations that can help change patterns of any illness, depression and bipolar disorder included, by recognizing negative beliefs and habits, and replacing them with new, positive beliefs that can transform your life.

Imagery

Mental imagery is also used to dispel recurring depression or flash-backs from traumatic experiences. For three decades Gerald Epstein, M.D., assistant clinical professor of psychiatry at New York's Mt. Sinai Medical Center, has taught how to use imagery to restore mental and physical health, and optimize one's potential.[2]

Dr. Epstein relates an experience with a chronically depressed woman. When asked to give an image that would describe her depression, she said, "The bottom of a pit." He asked that she see herself in the pit and then look around for something that would help her get out. She saw a rope ladder with hooks on the end and saw herself climbing the ladder out of the pit. At the top, she saw a wide-open space with light, sun, trees, and cows. When she opened her eyes, her depression was gone for the first time in thirteen years. She repeated the exercise to reinforce her decision to climb out of the pit and has remained depression-free.

Visual images are extremely powerful because they circumvent the logical mind through the use of mental pictures that are mediated through different areas of the brain. Instead of our rational mind maintaining the status quo, mental pictures show us an immediate vision of the change we want to make. The old sayings "A picture is worth a thousand words" and "Seeing is believing" are truisms reflecting how we react to images. For the mind, a vision is truth. According to Dr. Epstein, in his book *Healing Visualizations: Creating Health Through Imagery*, it normally takes twenty-one days of repetition for visualization to create change.

Yoga

I know from years of personal experience that a brisk thirty-minute walk is one of the easiest, fastest, and cheapest temporary remedies for mild depression. Exercise reduces stress and enhances overall metabolism, increasing the flow of oxygen and glucose to the brain. It promotes glucose use as well, stabilizing blood sugar levels, mood, and energy. Exercise raises serotonin levels, helps remove debris from brain cells, and boosts output of the neurotransmitters norepinephrine and dopamine.[3]

Yoga achieves similar effects through deep breathing, specific postures, and movement. Stimulation of the pituitary gland during yoga practice triggers the release of endorphins, hormones that promote a sense of well-being. Yoga dramatically reduces levels of the stress hormone cortisol after just one class.[4]

One small Scandinavian study measured brain waves before and after a two-hour yoga class, and found that the alpha waves of relaxed wakefulness and creativity and the theta waves of memory, dreams, and emotions were increased by 40 percent as a result of the yoga practice.[5] High levels of alpha waves indicate that we are "being" more than "doing," aware of the moment, in touch with our surroundings, mentally receptive.

The word *yoga* means "union" in Sanskrit, referring to the integration of mind, body, and spirit. For yoga is more than just exercise; it is a spiritual practice intended to increase one's receptivity to Universal energy, the life force called *prana*, *qi*, or *chi* (covered in the next chapter), which flows in through the chakras and which, over time, brings enlightenment.

In her 2004 book, *Yoga for Depression*, award-winning television producer and writer Amy Weintraub describes her recovery from depression in 1989 through daily yoga practice, covering the spiritual aspects and the traditions it entails. She discovered one breathing practice in particular, Sudarshan Kriya, that was responsible for a recovery rate as high as 73 percent among hospitalized patients suffering from major depression in India, comparing favorably to antidepressant medications.[6]

A 2005 report published by researchers at New York's Columbia College of Physicians and Surgeons states, "[T]here is sufficient evidence to consider Sudarshan Kriya Yoga to be a beneficial, low-risk, low-cost adjunct to the treatment of stress, anxiety, post-traumatic stress disorder, depression, . . ." The researchers recommended proper training by a skilled teacher and a thirty-minute practice every day to maximize benefits.[7]

Vibrations produced by chanting, used with some types of yoga, also have "a pronounced effect on our two most sensitive systems: the neurological and the endocrine [hormone]," according to Dharma Singh Khalsa, M.D., author of *Brain Longevity*. Chanting slows metabolism and heart rate, strengthens the vascular system, improves immune functioning, and increases brain-hemispheric balance.[8]

After a single yoga session, you feel calm, deeply relaxed, yet alert—the perfect state from which to meditate.

Meditation and Prayer

When unoccupied, the mind leaps and swings from thought to thought like a busy monkey. Meditation is concentration that quiets the active mind by focusing it on a singular thing in order to elicit a state of peace. Herbert Benson, M.D., founder of Harvard's Mind/ Body Medical Institute and one of the pioneers in the fields of behavioral medicine and mind/body studies, documented how meditation stimulates certain areas of the hypothalamus, affecting breathing rate, oxygen consumption, blood flow, and brain-wave rhythm.

According to Amy Weintraub, some types of meditation are better suited to certain mood disorders. She recommends mindfulness meditation, giving attention to the breath, for anxiety-based depression.[9] A 2001 study by the School of Psychology in Birmingham, England, explored mindfulness-based cognitive therapy for depression, finding that mindfulness skills "hold a key role in the development of change."[10]

Weintraub recommends zen meditation, where one focuses on breath or a riddle with no rational answer, as a way to interrupt obsessive thought patterns, and transcendental meditation, which uses repetition of a mantra, for calming. A research group at the Institute for Nonlinear Science in San Diego found kundalini yoga best for treating obsessive-compulsive disorder.[11]

Prayer is sometimes considered mind/body communion, a type of meditation, and an alternative therapy. In a report on complementary and alternative medicine (CAM) use in 2002 among 31,004 adults in the United States, when prayer for health reasons was included in the definition of CAM, 62 percent were said to use "complementary therapies." When prayer was excluded from the definition, the figure dropped to only 36 percent use.[12]

Is prayer therapeutic? A review article in the *Journal of the American Geriatrics Society* in 2000, citing an international study of 170,000 men and women in fourteen countries, found religious affiliation and attendance at houses of worship significantly increased the likelihood of happiness and satisfaction. A Yale Health and Aging Study, drawing on twelve years of data, showed that, on average, members of religious congregations had slower onset of physical disability.[13]

Researchers in Victoria, Australia, did controlled studies of the benefits of incorporating spirituality into psychological therapy. They found "16-session spiritually augmented cognitive behavioural therapy to be beneficial in extinguishing hopelessness and despair, improving treatment collaboration, reducing relapse rates, and enhancing functional recovery."[14] Yes, prayer is therapeutic, and so are your other beliefs.

The "placebo effect" is an improvement in health that arises from a patient's expectations, rather than from the treatment itself. Established by Dr. Henry K. Beecher of Massachusetts General Hospital in a 1955 study as roughly 30 percent of the healing, that percentage is still what drugs and therapies strive to beat today, proving they are more effective than a person's belief.

Dr. Herbert Benson explored this further at Harvard's Mind/Body Medical Institute in the mid-1970s. He tracked the contribution of a person's desire for health and the human body's propensity to turn the individual's beliefs into a physical instruction and found it even more powerful—70–90 percent effective.[15]

Doctors and drug companies often say something is "merely the placebo effect," but to me, there is nothing *mere* about 70–90 percent. The placebo effect is, in fact, one of the most powerful medicines! Mind/body integration and energy medicines harness this amazing innate capability and use it for self-healing.

Carolyn Myss, in *Anatomy of the Spirit*, writes, "You alone can help yourself heal." The process of *curing* is passive: The patient is inclined to give his or her authority over to the physician or treatment. "*Healing*, on the other hand, is an active and internal process that includes investigating one's attitudes, memories, and beliefs with the desire to release all negative patterns that prevent one's full emotional and spiritual recovery."[16]

CHAPTER 12

Energy Healing: Therapeutic Touch, Reiki, and Acupuncture

Lindsae Raineau developed suicidal depression at age thirteen. Her family had recently moved and did not notice her withdrawal. "I alienated myself from the family. I either wanted to be alone or with my friends, and I started hiding out in my room a lot, writing poetry," recalls the young woman.

Most parents would consider this normal teenage behavior, but Lindsae's problems went deeper. "I had issues with my father, and I didn't know whether there was an underlying problem or whether it was because I only saw him once a year." How did she know this wasn't just normal teenage, hormonal mood swings? "I was having a lot harder time coping than my friends. I had always really been care-free and happy, and I didn't like that I was losing the zest for life that was normally a part of me," she explains.

Lindsae's mother felt the blues would blow over, but when the teenager confided that she was seriously struggling and having thoughts of suicide, she was immediately placed in therapy. Diagnosed with depression and put on Prozac, then Zoloft, the teenager improved, but was "not happy with the idea of taking drugs to make myself feel better. I just wanted a different approach."

Jill Adams, a therapeutic touch practitioner in Mystic, Connecticut, had helped Lindsae's mother and suggested that Lindsae try it for depression.[1] "I was very skeptical, not really sure what to expect,"

Lindsae recalls. "It was kind of a leap of faith. I was willing to try any-thing."

Lindsae went to see Jill weekly at first; then, as she became more stable, every two weeks. By accessing Lindsae's personal energy field (explained later), the therapist was able to impact the teenager's mood and physical energy. "Jill helped me work through issues I knew were there but that hadn't come to a head yet. I always felt very calm and at peace when I left. So, I kept going back."

Through gentle massage and touch, Jill "worked on releasing dif-ferent areas of the body where I hold certain energy," says Lindsae. "Working with her kept me grounded, bringing me back to myself and not letting me get caught up in everything that was making me depressed."

The two talked as well. "I think I was learning to be aware of how I fit into the world, but I don't really know how to explain that," Lind-sae says, laughing. "I had a lot of conflict with my mother growing up. Jill and I would talk about that and she would make suggestions about how to handle a situation.

"I feel working with Jill made me a more spiritual person. She gave me a different perspective on my place in the world and how the de-cisions I make affect other people and how other people's decisions affect me. Every time I walked out after a session, I would definitely feel lighter, like a weight had been lifted. Generally, I would feel that way for a couple of days. Every session with Jill, I would get a little bit better."

Lindsae moved frequently as a child and now became aware that any major change triggered depression. "As I grew older," she recalls, "I came to realize that I could somehow control this, by doing yoga or going to sessions with Jill, or just taking myself out of a situation and thinking about it."

Lindsae had taken antibiotics frequently for childhood ear infec-tions and chronic illnesses; a naturopathic physician now found that she had candida yeast overgrowth. She began using antifungal med-ications, detoxification, and diet to rid herself of the yeast and lift her moods. An athlete who was raised to be aware of the impact of foods, Lindsae experienced such a "life-altering" improvement from the candida reduction diet that she continues following a modified version of it today.

The doctor also suggested that she start taking amino acids. "I felt so much more alert, not nearly as depressed. Fatigue is something I've always struggled with too, and I felt much better with the combination of diet and amino acids together."

When Lindsae began college, she found a job working in a bar. Both the diet and amino acids were soon forgotten. She experimented with drugs and alcohol, quickly learning that the next morning her depression was "ten times worse" than it had been the night before. On her own for the first time, she "was partying five days a week, just out of control. I kind of crashed. When I started looking into a mirror and really hating myself, I realized I had a problem with alcohol, and I couldn't continue like that.

"The drugs I was trying and the people I was hanging out with— the whole scene was just so dark that I was, like, this isn't what I want for myself." Although rejecting drugs quickly, alcohol continued to be a challenge. "Even now when I drink socially, the next day I have the blues, so I just try and stay away from it."

Once she became aware of how her associates and her social environment contributed to her depression, she decided to try making a change. Lindsae and a girlfriend moved one summer to San Diego, a place where she had always wanted to live, consciously cutting out of her life negative people, places, and substances. "I went through my phase of depression, again, because I was in a new setting and afraid. But I got a job, found a place to live, and it was actually great because I realized I could do it on my own."

At summer's end, Lindsae returned to Mystic while finishing college. Her mother, meanwhile, was studying to become a certified reflexologist. Reflexology is an ancient practice that involves manipulating points on the bottom and tops of the feet to release toxins and break up energy blockages in the body. Needing someone to practice on, her mother worked on Lindsae, who experienced what this therapy did for her moods. "I always had anxiety too, not just depression. I found that reflexology had a relaxing effect that helped my anxiety."

While finishing her degree in behavioral science, Lindsae worked briefly at a transitional living facility for women and children who had been abused. "A lot of times I was feeling depressed because of problems they were having," she says. Realizing that she became too emotionally involved for a career in this field, she explored other options.

Today, Lindsae is a vibrant twenty-six-year-old mother who works with Health in Harmony, where she is putting together a detoxification program for autistic children, incorporating the far infrared sauna treatment with massage and her own Touch for Health practice.

To avoid slipping into depression, she takes vitamins and watches her diet, avoiding sugars and carbohydrates, while trying to eat natural, organic foods without preservatives. She also strives to fit some kind of exercise into her schedule five days a week.

Lindsae's experience is a coming-of-age saga for emotionally sensitive teenagers. Learning which ups and downs are driven by hormones, physical ailments, or life situations, while building self-confidence and self-awareness, is a big challenge, but not an insurmountable one, given the right guidance and a bit of determination.

Energy Medicines

In *Vibrational Medicine*, Richard Gerber, M.D., states, "Quantum physics and experiments in high-energy particle physics have shown us that, at the particle level, all matter is really energy. If we are beings of energy, then it follows that we can be affected by energy."[2] His book offers a comprehensive history of energetic medicine, from its beginnings through its evolution, explaining the various methods.

Jill Adams, the woman who helped Lindsae, uses a form of energy medicine called therapeutic touch or hands-on healing. In a

2005 study designed to evaluate the effectiveness of gentle touch (as it is called in England), three hundred subjects with a wide range of ailments received four treatments within six weeks. Outcome was measured by comparing pre- and post-treatment levels of physical functioning (pain, disability, immobility, sleep disturbances, reliance on medication, daily activities) and psychological functioning (stress, panic, fear, anger, relaxation, coping, depression/anxiety). Statistically significant improvements were found in both psychological and physical functioning, particularly in stress reduction, pain relief, and increased ability to cope. "The most substantial improvements were seen in those with the most severe symptoms at study entry."[3]

Therapeutic touch, reiki, acupuncture, and numerous other types of energy medicine all work by enhancing the flow of subtle energies in the body and aura. The aura is a multilayered energy field resembling a bubble that extends beyond a human's physical body three or more feet. Surrounding and penetrating each living entity, it is protective and nurturing, filtering out some energies and drawing in others needed through a system of chakras (discussed later).[4] Subtle energies form a light-blue or gray outline around the body, sometimes visible by squinting your eyes as you view a person in bright light. Outside this fuzzy outline are other layers of color comprising the aura (visible to psychics but not to most other people).

Increasing the flow of a person's subtle energies was seldom discussed in the United States until the 1960s. However, it has been studied and practiced by other cultures for millennia to help achieve physical or emotional healing and to aid in spiritual growth. Five-thousand-year-old Indian spiritual traditions called such energy *prana*. The Chinese named it *chi* in the third millennium B.C. The Kabbalah, the book of Jewish mysticism, refers to it as astral light. Ancient Hindu Vedic texts, theosophists, Rosicrucians, Native American shamans, Tibetan and Indian Buddhists, and Japanese Zen Buddhists all recognize human energy fields.

The very idea was long scoffed at by scientific America because the energies couldn't be seen by most or measured. During the 1940s, however, tangible evidence of the auras' existence was found. Neuroanatomist Harold S. Burr was studying electrical fields surrounding salamanders at Yale University when he determined that the amphibians possessed an energy field roughly shaped like the adult animal and that it contained an electrical axis aligned with the brain and spinal cord. By mapping the fields in progressively earlier stages of embryogenesis, he discovered that they originated in the unfertilized egg. Subsequent experiments using tiny seedlings showed that the surrounding energy field resembled the adult plant, suggesting that the aura was a template for growth generated by an organism's individual electromagnetic field.[5]

Russian researcher Semyon Kirlian, working around the same time, developed a method of photographing living objects in the presence of high-frequency, high-voltage, low-amperage electrical fields, capturing a view of their aura. Both men's techniques for measuring the aura added physical proof of its existence and later demonstrated that many diseases, like cancer, caused significant changes in both the color and shape of the aura, opening the door for using the aura in diagnosis.[6]

Another favorite resource that explains energy healing is Barbara A. Brennan's *Hands of Light: A Guide to Healing Through the Human Energy Field*.[7] A former NASA research scientist who became a hands-on healer, Barbara founded the Barbara Brennan School of Healing in Florida, which has become the preeminent energy healing training center.[8] Barbara describes seven layers of the aura that receive energy through the chakras from the larger Universal field that interconnects all living things. Humans are more than just living in a "global village"; it seems we are all connected energetically.

Energy flows into the body through seven major invisible, funnel-shaped vortices, called chakras. Each chakra is aligned with significant nerve centers, glands, and organs. Chakras have three major functions: (1) to vitalize each aura and, thus, the physical body; (2) to bring about development of self-consciousness, each vortex having specific psychological functions; and (3) to transmit energy between auric levels (the layers of colors), with "higher" levels opening as a result of greater spiritual growth and purification.

In simple terms, blockage of energy within the body creates conditions that prevent our innate physical healing mechanisms from working, thus eventually causing all disease. The body has built-in methods to kill bacteria and viruses, to eliminate toxins, or to stop mutant cells from proliferating, but these systems are impeded by energy blockages. Releasing blockages to restore natural health by improving the flow of Universal life energy is a fascinating new field (at least to us).

Therapeutic touch, reiki, acupuncture, and massage therapy are being used in many hospitals for one reason: Doctors have learned that they do reduce pain, increase postoperative healing, and ease depression, anxiety, and stress, although medical professionals don't yet fully understand just how these practices work.[9] Some practitioners predict that energy therapies will become the dominant healing modality of the twenty-first century, replacing drugs and surgery as surely as those methods replaced bleeding and leeches.

The function of major chakras, their associated colors, and the areas of the body affected by them are spelled out in the box.

MAJOR CHAKRAS	COLOR	BODY AREAS AFFECTED
#1 Root	Red	Spinal column, Kidneys
#2 Sacral	Orange	Gonads, Reproductive system
#3 Solar Plexus	Yellow	Adrenals, Digestive and Detoxification organs, Nervous system
#4 Heart	Green	Thymus, Heart, Blood, Circulatory System
#5 Throat	Sky Blue	Thyroid, Respiratory and Vocal system

#6 Head	Indigo	Pituitary, Lower brain, Left eye, Ears, Nose, Autonomic nervous system
#7 Crown	Violet/White	Upper brain, Right eye, Central nervous system

Energy from chakras is delivered throughout the body by a network of meridians, fourteen tangible pathways that carry energy to all major organs and physiological systems. Since meridians corresponded to no known anatomical structures, they were also disputed in the West until the 1960s, when injection of radioactive isotopes into acupuncture points demonstrated the existence of an intricate network having fine ductlike tubules approximately 0.5–1.5 micron in diameter that followed ancient descriptions of meridian pathways.[10] The energy flowing through meridians is accessed at acupuncture points to release or redistribute energy.

Acupuncture

Part of Chinese medicine for three thousand years, acupuncture is based on the belief that health is determined by balancing the flow of *chi* (also called *qi*) along the meridians. Manipulating the flow of energy is done by inserting fine needles (or using heat, pressure, friction, suction, or impulses of electromagnetic energy) into specific points in the body, called acupoints.

Chinese immigrants brought acupuncture to this country in the mid-1800s, but American doctors didn't become intrigued by the practice until 1972, when a respected *New York Times* columnist, James Reston, underwent an emergency appendectomy while in China and reported the amazing pain relief he gained from acupuncture.[11]

Researchers working under a grant from the National Institutes of Health soon proved that electrical currents did flow along the meridians and that 25 percent of acupuncture points did exist, speculating that these points act as amplifiers that could be used to boost or block minute electrical signals, thus interrupting pain.

As knowledge of acupuncture's benefits spread, counselors in substance-abuse programs in the United States discovered that acupuncture treatments reduced drug use by as much as 50 percent (and reduced reincarceration rates in a group of women prisoners by 26 percent). By 1995, there were approximately three hundred acupuncture-based substance-abuse programs in this country.[12] This, of course, indicates that acupuncture is beneficial for brain chemistry disorders, but recent clinical trials using acupuncture for depression have shown inconclusive results, attributed to the complexity of designing such studies.[13]

Reiki

Funding for clinical trials of all alternative therapies was nonexistent until consumer demand—and the cost of prescription drugs—made it a recent government priority. Thus, I was surprised to find a 2004 study of forty-six depressed participants who used reiki for at least one hour a week for six weeks. The outcome—measured by the Beck Depression Inventory, Beck Hopelessness, and Perceived Stress scales—showed a significant reduction in symptoms of psychological distress, as compared with controls, and the differences were still pronounced a year later.[14]

Reiki (pronounced RAY-key) is a Japanese word meaning universal life. The healing practice was developed by Mikao Usui, who was born in Japan in 1864 and raised by Christian missionaries. After studying the Bible and learning of Jesus' acts of healing, Usui became a theology professor and was appointed head of a Christian boys' school. One morning, several of the boys asked if he literally believed in the biblical miracles Jesus performed. He replied that he did. The boys challenged him to demonstrate his faith by performing a miracle.

Dr. Usui's search to understand how such miracles were achieved spanned seven years in America studying scripture, a return to Japan, and several more years at a monastery studying and meditating on Buddhist scriptures. Within ancient Sanskrit texts, he discovered the symbols that led him to the healing techniques that comprise reiki practice today.[15] Dr. Usui discovered how to access the Universal energy surrounding all of us and use it for healing.

After training, reiki practitioners receive four empowerments (or attunements) that open up subtle mental and physical energy systems, and prepare them to channel Universal life force energy. After the fourth attunement, reiki energy is established within the practitioner's energy system for life, available for personal use or to aid others. Reiki flows from the hands of the therapist, impacting the energy of any living organism—be it a human being, another animal, or a plant.

If I had read about reiki before using it, I probably would not have tried it. The whole concept simply sounds too incredible. Fortunately, I was treated first.

Stung on my lower back by a wasp one night, I was too groggy to make a baking soda paste to draw out the venom (an old trick from my beekeeping father). By morning, the poison had moved throughout my spine and I was in agony. I went to Stonebridge Herbary in Mystic looking for natural pain relief.[16] The owner, Bonnie Rogers, said, "Why don't you let me do some reiki on it. It'll only take ten minutes." I had never heard of reiki, but Bonnie was always a reliable healing resource. After the treatment, the spot where I had been stung felt warm. That was all. By morning, I had no pain anywhere.

Therapeutic Touch

Years ago I had little knowledge of energy healing when I tried it for my bipolar cycles. At that point, treatments at the Pfeiffer Center had resolved my mania but I was still suffering from depression. Reiki had proven effective for a temporary ailment, and I had since read Barbara

Brennan's books. Would "energy balancing" help control my depression? I did not believe or disbelieve, I simply opened my mind enough to give it a try.

From the first session, I felt tingling sensations in my body, had a sense of peace, and saw colors and shapes flash behind closed eyelids as Ellie Brown, the Barbara Brennan–trained healer I used, gently touched my arm and began moving energy through my body.[17] These subtle reactions indicated to me that *something* was happening, although I had no idea what. After six months of one-hour weekly energy-balancing sessions, Ellie said my blockages were cleared and my energy was balanced, but she was a bit puzzled about why my energy wouldn't remain balanced.

This is when I learned to pay close attention to intriguing "coincidences" that Deepak Chopra, M.D., a celebrated author, says increase when you use meditation or energy work (in his wonderful book *The Spontaneous Fulfillment of Desire: Harnessing the Infinite Power of Coincidence*).[18] After I had done everything I could think of to permanently lift my depression without apparent success, the most amazing coincidence occurred.

A total stranger, Lawrence G., telephoned me to check the references of Pfeiffer Treatment Center for a family member stuck in mania. Although I had authorized the clinic to give out my name and number, this was the first person to call in fifteen months. I told Lawrence the center had quickly eliminated my mania but had not eradicated my depression. He told me about Dr. Andrew Stoll's book *The Omega-3 Connection*, and the author's successful use of fish oils with bipolar patients.

I began taking the oils immediately, my depression lifted within forty-eight hours, and at my next appointment with Ellie, she said, "What are you doing different? Your energy is the best I've seen in anyone in a very long time." My energy has stayed in balance ever since.

It took a couple more years before I understood that what had happened to me was a classic example of how energy healing often works. Practitioners remove blockages and correct the impeded flow of energy that, over time, compromises physical and emotional well-being. Then, through remarkable synchronicities, the door to physical wellness simply opens up—in my case, as a result of a total stranger calling me from Kentucky with information about fish oils that enabled healing on the physical level and maintaining balanced energy.

Energy medicine refers to therapies that utilize Universal energy to correct illnesses in numerous ways, including acupuncture, acupressure, aromatherapy, craniosacral manipulation, hands-on healing, Hellinger therapy, kinesiology, light or sound therapy, magnetic field therapy, medical intuitive diagnosis, reiki, reflexology, *qi qong*, therapeutic touch, yoga, and the subject of the next chapter, homeopathy.

CHAPTER 13

Homeopathy: A Potent Medical System

No one would ever suspect that Suzy, a slender, dynamic mortgage broker with short brown hair and hazel eyes, had suffered from anxiety and suicidal depression for twenty years as a result of childhood sexual abuse by her stepfather. Although outwardly successful, she was adversely affected by the abuse, which had an impact on every aspect of her life.

Suzy's first two marriages ended in divorce. Her third husband was "needy," and as stress in the relationship increased, she began to develop severe hives all over her body. A psychologist in the clinic where she was working at the time asked what was going on in her life.

"There's a whole lot of stress in my life, and I don't think I'm dealing with it very well," Suzy responded. Her doctor placed her on Zoloft, and the hives immediately disappeared.

Suzy entered counseling, and for nine months worked to deal with the childhood abuse, using a combination of regression under hypnotherapy, talk therapy, and Zoloft. "It made a huge difference in my life," she recalls. "I was able to talk it out with my stepfather and there came a point where I was able to forgive him." After two years, she gradually went off Zoloft, feeling she didn't need it anymore.

Years later, Suzy had a partial hysterectomy that triggered early menopause and a return of the depression. Now working in the high-pressure mortgage industry and still struggling with the marriage, she was even more stressed and had trouble sleeping. "I'd wake up three or four times during the night, thinking about work, financial stuff, pressures, trying to figure out how to take care of things," she says. "Many nights it seemed like I was awake all night."

"My mom—who suffered childhood sexual abuse as well and helped me with the cost of my initial therapy—had sleep disturbances when she was in her forties too. She had treated herself with sleeping pills and had a terrible time getting off them, for ten, twelve years or more, so I will not allow myself to get dependent on medications."

Suzy's hives returned, making her tongue and her entire face swell up. When touched, she bruised. "I looked like I had been beaten up. My body just reacts physically to stress." She went back on Zoloft for a year before tapering off, trying to avoid drug dependency.

Within a short time, "I knew I was falling into the deep hole of depression again." Says Suzy, "I was very emotional but not able to let go and cry. I had no sex drive. I wasn't able to dream. I just felt like I was in a pit and couldn't get out. There was no light." Unable to afford more therapy, this time she decided to try a different approach.

After filing for divorce in 2003, she joined a business referral group and met Tim Shannon, a naturopathic doctor with a decade of experience using homeopathy to treat schizophrenia and bipolar disorder at a Portland, Oregon, mental health clinic. He also treated HIV/AIDS homeopathically, helping to open a clinic in Kenya.

In November 2003, Dr. Shannon interviewed Suzy for about an hour, videotaping the session. Homeopathic remedies are selected based on the patient's personality traits, idiosyncrasies, preferences, phobias, and symptoms, attempting to match these variables to one precise remedy (explained in more detail later). Dr. Shannon prescribed an exceedingly rare plant-based homeopathic formula because of Suzy's specific indications and his success with some of its botanical relatives.

"It took me several weeks to notice a very gradual, subtle change," says Suzy. "Within two months, I was able to cry. I started going back to my home church and was able to *feel* what I was going through and express those emotions." The depression became "lighter," but her hives got worse and she still awoke several times a night. Dr. Shannon increased her dosage.

By April, the hives were subsiding, but when she was out of town without her homeopathic medicine, they came back. The good news she gave the doctor was this: "I am sleeping! I don't do anything special, and I sleep until six or seven. I'm dreaming—I can't remember my dreams, but realize I'm dreaming. My confidence is coming back. Life is just a lot righter. There is still a lot of stress, but I'm managing it better. I don't feel like I'm in that deep dark pit anymore."

After fifteen months, Suzy's depression was totally gone and she seldom had hives. Of the twelve symptoms she complained of during their first interview, half had been completely resolved and the other half had improved under the homeopathic regimen.

Homeopathy also allowed Suzy to avoid becoming dependent on any medications. Whenever stresses started to become overwhelming again, she would call Dr. Shannon for more of the remedy, but she has not had to do so for almost a year.

When a person's depression has lifted, she has energy to deal with other physical problems and *consistently* do things that support overall health. Suzy began taking good-quality multivitamins, using the natural relaxant Formula 303[1] when she was especially stressed and taking Ageless Extra[2] once or twice a day to promote cellular regeneration. She started walking or running three to four times a week. "I'm trying to take care of my physical body as well as my mental health," she explains.

To release the tension[3] stored in her neck and back, Suzy consulted Kirsten Hope,[4] a hypnotherapist and practitioner of BodyTalk, a healing system developed by John Veltheim, D.C. Former academic chair of the Australian Chiropractic Association and principal director for the College of Chinese Medicine and Natural Therapies in Brisbane, Dr. Veltheim used the practices he incorporated into BodyTalk to bring himself back from the brink of death, eliminating chronic Epstein-Barr virus and a high fever that lasted six years.

BodyTalk includes elements of advanced yoga, advaitic philosophy, physics, mathematics, acupuncture, kinesiology, and Western medicine to access the body's innate wisdom. Using a comprehensive list of questions, a practitioner can "resynchronize" the mind/body function by means of tapping and touch. Suzy was able to isolate stressful situations by using specific tapping points. The method has also proven successful for musculoskeletal problems (sports injuries, back problems, arthritis), detoxification, activating immune response to chronic viruses and infections, and learning or behavioral disorders.

Just three sessions made an impact for Suzy. "One time was to get all my *chi* in line and key into my adrenal glands—that made a huge difference. Two visits eliminated muscle stuff going on in my shoulders and upper back." Several acupuncture treatments augmented the BodyTalk sessions.

In just three hypnotherapy sessions, she was able to reduce procrastination and other negative traits she felt were holding her back. Suzy then made rapid progress, developing an idea that would solve a health care need she noticed while caring for a quadriplegic neighbor.

Paralyzed and nonambulatory people go through painful bowel procedures, sitting on commode chairs with little padding, sometimes for two to three hours at a time, three to four times a week. To reduce their pain and possible pressure sores, Suzy created a commode chair cushion, which evolved into about eight other types of seats. She patented the cushions within six months and formed her own corporation, OADES Products, specializing in items that help those in wheelchairs and the elderly. "I'm getting more excited about my career change and new venture," she says with pride and anticipation. "It's a major shift in my life, and a lot of that is due to homeopathy getting me out of the depression so I could move forward."

Homeopathy's Promise

Homeopathy is the ideal therapy for bipolar children or anyone too depressed, young, violent, or paranoid to assist much with their own healing. Homeopathic remedies are simple, inexpensive (generally ranging from $7 to $20), and can be used in conjunction with psychiatric medications until symptoms are sufficiently under control to eliminate the drugs. In the hands of a skilled practitioner, this approach requires no special diet, no vitamin/mineral supplements, and almost no effort by a patient, other than taking the homeopathic fluids daily.

Impossible Cure: The Promise of Homeopathy by Amy L. Lansky, Ph.D., explains in detail just how it works. A former computer science researcher for NASA and a consulting associate professor at Stanford, Lansky skillfully interweaves details about this unusual, even counterintuitive, medical approach with the moving saga of how it cured her autistic son.[5]

Homeopathy was created in 1796 by Christian Frederich Samuel Hahnemann in Meissen, Germany. Fluent in German, English, French, Italian, Latin, and Greek and able to translate Hebrew, Chaldaic, and Arabic, he began medical studies at age twenty, augmenting his income by translating scientific texts.

Dr. Hahnemann soon found the medical practices of his time—induced sweating, vomiting, diarrhea; bleeding through vein cutting or application of leeches; sedating with opiates; and using toxic doses of mercury—of questionable value. By age twenty-nine, he concluded that a doctor's best option was to follow one of Hippocrates's lesser-known directives (the famed one for all physicians is "First, do no harm"): Intensely observe patients' symptoms by sitting at their bedside and assist their healing only with natural techniques, such as diet, good hygiene, and improved living conditions.

Dr. Hahnemann became more outspoken in his criticism of orthodox medical practices. Then, as today, medicine was big business, and he paid dearly for challenging the medical establishment of his day. Opening a practice in Hettstedt, he soon became an itinerant physician, often ridiculed and run out of town by the pharmacists because he prepared his own medicines and threatened their livelihood. He relocated his family at least eighteen times between 1782 and 1821.[6]

Finally, he temporarily gave up his medical practice to translate prestigious medical and scientific texts, for which he was highly regarded. The dawn of homeopathy came while Dr. Hahnemann was translating the *Treatise on Materia Medica* in 1790. Its author, William Cullen, a professor of medicine at the University of Edinburgh, described the use of *cinchona* (a Peruvian bark that was the wonder drug of the eighteenth century) for malaria, attributing its success to a tonic effect on the stomach, which made no sense to the translator.

Dr. Hahnemann recalled that Hippocrates maintained that a cure could best be achieved through the actions of "opposites," using a medicine that creates an effect opposite that of the patient's symptoms, or through the action of "similars," using one that creates the same symptoms in a *healthy* individual. He decided to put the latter hypothesis to a test, using himself as a guinea pig. Taking *cinchona* for several days, he induced symptoms of malaria that ceased when the medicine was discontinued.

Such testing of substances, later called *provings*, became Dr. Hahnemann's life work and a pillar of his medical approach, which he called *homeoeopathy*—meaning "similar suffering." According to his "Law of Similars," a substance that causes, in a healthy person, symptoms similar to those of a disease state, can cure a sick person in that disease state.[7]

Homeopathy's popularity grew rapidly—largely due to its superior results. The very first medical association of any kind in the United States was the American Institute of Homeopathy, founded in 1844, two years before the American Medical Association. The first woman's medical college was also homeopathic, the New England Female Medical College, founded in 1848.[8] In the nineteenth century, there were more than twenty homeopathic medical schools in this country. Advocated by the wealthy, presidents, politicians, and the armed forces, homeopathy soon threatened allopathy, or conventional medicine.

By the mid-1800s, allopathic doctors had organized and expelled or barred homeopathic practitioners from their societies, periodicals, and pharmacies. The American Medical Association's growing power received a boost in the early 1900s through the introduction of aspirin, antibiotics, x-rays, and vaccinations, faster-acting medicines that made allopathy more financially lucrative than homeopathy. By 1950, there were only one hundred homeopathic physicians still practicing in this country, although the practice remained popular abroad.

During the 1970s, several young San Francisco Bay Area doctors, frustrated by conventional medicine's inability to cure chronic diseases, resuscitated its use. Today, homeopathy is enjoying a renaissance, with homeopathic medicines offered by medical doctors, naturopathic doctors, osteopaths, chiropractors, acupuncturists, and professional homeopaths, specifically trained and certified by the Council for Homeopathic Certification (CHC) and the North American Society of Homeopaths (NASH). Doctors with three years of homeopathic practice may seek board certification and, if successful, affix the designation D.Ht. after their name.

Homeopathic treatments are made from all-natural mineral, plant, or animal substances, highly diluted with water through a process called *potentization*. The primary argument used against homeopathy has always been that the medicines are so diluted that, from a biochemical standpoint, they no longer contain a single molecule of the original substance. Thus, according to conventional science, they cannot possibly work. However, they have proven safe and effective for two hundred years and are regulated today by the FDA as a drug, using the Homeopathic Pharmacopoeia of the United States (HPUS) as the official compendium of standards.[9]

Today most practitioners believe that the homeopathic potentization process in some way "charges" the water used to dilute it, imbuing it with the energy of the natural substance, which in turn activates the body's energy field, triggering a healing response. Since all forms of energy medicine are perched on the cutting edge of tomorrow's science, homeopathic treatment will be debated for years to come. Thanks to its history of success and the very low cost of homeopathic treatments, it is enjoying a resurgence of use.

Since studies of homeopathy's effectiveness are small, meta-analysis is an ideal way to measure whether or not the results are real or "only a placebo effect." Meta-analysis is a process that uses collective data from diverse clinical trials to study one phenomenon. First reported in the *British Medical Journal* in 1988 and considered a breakthrough, meta-analysis was the method used to determine that taking a daily aspirin helped prevent heart attacks. Two meta-analyses of homeopathy, one published in 1991 and another in 1997, both demonstrated that the effects of homeopathic medicines clearly exceed those of placebos. The 1997 study, published in *The Lancet*, a respected British medical journal, found that homeopathy was nearly 250 percent more effective than a placebo, an impressive finding, considering that the much-heralded 1988 meta-analysis of aspirin showed that it was merely 75 percent more effective than a placebo.[10]

The controversy in the research world, sparked by the 1997 study, is still raging. One positive effect of the ongoing conflict between advocates and opponents of homeopathy is that it has triggered a flurry of additional homeopathic trials, seeking to confirm or disprove the 1997 study.

A 2003 homeopathy trial showed "statistically significant results in subjects with stage III AIDS," as well as specific physical, immunological, neurological, metabolic, and quality-of-life benefits, including improved lymphocyte counts and reductions in HIV viral loads.[11] A 2004 study of homeopathy for patients with fibromyalgia showed "that individualized homeopathy is significantly better than placebo in lessening tender point pain."[12]

There is one fundamental difference between homeopathic and conventional allopathic medicine: the approach. Allopathic medicine looks at problems in isolation, intently focusing on an area or organ where a symptom appears. The dizzying rate of discovery in the medical world has splintered conventional medicine into an array of specialists, each only knowledgeable about her own field, leaving no one looking at the whole. Patients end up taking twelve different medications, which often have adverse interactions, all offering perpetual *treatment* but seldom a cure, while making for unpredictable long-term side effects.

Dr. Hahnemann found that if *all* of a patient's traits and symptoms were initially considered and treated with *one* homeopathic remedy—the right one—the patient would be cured and experience no further disease progression. As a result, *classical* homeopathy still uses only one remedy at a time. Having over 1,600 to choose from, practitioners spend hours learning the details of a patient's personality along with his symptoms (as Dr. Shannon did in taped interviews with Suzy), then do extensive research to find the specific remedy that may bring about a cure: complete restoration of health so that no further medicine is needed.

Selecting a well-trained and experienced homeopathic practitioner is vital to success. If you do not know someone who can recommend a practitioner, consult the Web (www.homeopathyhome.com; www.homeopathicdirectory.com, sponsored by the Council for Homeopathic Certification; and www.homeopathy-cures.com/html/referrals_to_homeopaths.html), a site hosted by the president of the North American Society of Homeopaths, Steve Waldstein, and his wife Aviva, both practicing classical homeopaths.

PART III

Creating Your Future

CHAPTER 14

Restoring Mental Health

Tracy Boudreau called me in January 2005 after picking up a flier for my natural healing seminar at a health food store. She was bipolar, a single mother, and on disability, so could not afford the fee and asked if I offered scholarships. As the forty-two-year-old told me her story, she struggled to be matter-of-fact, but I could hear the desperation in her voice.

"My mother was manic-depressive," said Tracy, "and I was born into a family full of addiction and riddled with violence. I was twelve years old when I started having symptoms. I remember clearly one of the school counselors saying, 'Gosh, Tracy, we never know until we see you in the morning what kind of day it's going to be. You're an absolute emotional roller coaster.'"

That year, Tracy made her first suicide attempt, one of several in her early teens. "I was depressed and crying and decided I wanted to die. We had a very large picture window in our living room, I took both fists and all my body weight, and I hit the window." She was lucky, suffering only cuts and lacerations on her head and arms.

Living on her own by the age of fifteen, Tracy recalls the first time she was institutionalized. "I was a young, single mother, living in Chicago. I hadn't been able to afford any type of Christmas for me or my son, and I became severely depressed." Sitting alone in her apartment, she took a large kitchen knife and started making small cuts on her arm for perhaps an hour. "Then I just lost it, and in a flash I took that knife and hacked at my arm three times." The damage required roughly fifty stitches that, along with a bloody apartment, drew the attention of her family and state officials.

Tracy's father placed her in an exceptional hospital in a Chicago suburb that said they could help her. "I remember thinking, 'Oh, thank God, finally. Somebody knows what's wrong with me and can fix it,'" says Tracy. When the hospital discovered that her father had long ago canceled his insurance coverage for Tracy, however, she was asked to leave.

Due to the severity of her suicide attempt, doctors wanted to place Tracy in the state mental hospital. "I refused, and they set me up with outpatient therapy. My sister took care of my son, but I was a mess and had no transportation. I would have to use all these trains and buses to get there to talk to this woman. I think I went once or twice. The help they were offering was too difficult. When you're that depressed, just getting up and out of the house is difficult."

Later, Tracy took an overdose of street drugs, walked in front of cars, and even prayed that God would kill her in an accident. Says Tracy, "I don't know if there is any way to tell someone who has never experienced suicidal thoughts just how devastating and horrible and complete that void is. It takes over your every emotion, everything that you love. It's stronger than anything else, and it's a deep, black abyss. It swallows you," she says. "When I go through episodes of suicidal behavior and feelings, it's total blackness. The emotional pain is so horrible and it's constant. It's in your brain, so there's no avoiding it. Death seems better. It truly feels like the only option."

As the years went by, Tracy's doctors tried seventeen different psychiatric drugs and combinations. None helped. She underwent electroconvulsive therapy. "I begged the doctors to give it to me. I had tried many therapies and every drug imaginable, and I was getting worse. I read about electroshock therapy and thought, 'This is it!' I was so desperate, I would have done anything." It left her brain "like mush," wiping out her short-term and long-term memory, and causing this articulate woman to grope for simple words. It did not, however, diminish the suicidal urges.

Tracy was not the only one in her family to find death appealing. "My sister, Kathy, was a brilliant scientist and very successful. She truly believed that some type of medicine would cure her. Suicidal through most of her adult life, at the end she became self-destructive, going to several different doctors and pharmacies to get all the medications she believed would help her. In June of 2000, she put a handgun in her mouth and blew her head off.

"My mother was very smart, very funny, and absolutely beautiful. She was also a violent alcoholic, and I'm sure that was directly related to her bipolar disorder. She was Irish and would get very excited about holidays. For St. Patty's Day, she would dye everything green—the ice cubes, the mashed potatoes—and paint four-leaf clovers on our faces with green food coloring," Tracy says, laughing. "Before a holiday, the excitement would build and build—her mania, unknown to us at the time. Inevitably, she would destroy every holiday she had put so much energy into, drunkenly knocking over the Christmas tree or having bloody fights with my father. She drank herself to death in 2001.

"My son, a deeply sensitive poet, was also severely depressed. They must have started him on psychiatric drugs at age five. When he left home at sixteen, he went from prescriptions to street drugs. He told me that as much as he hated heroin and how it was destroying his life, nothing felt so beautiful, calmed him down, and made him feel like everything was okay like heroin. He used a dirty needle, contracted AIDS and hepatitis C, then developed a brain tumor and died in 2003."

Several times as we talked, Tracy told me how her daughter, Stephanie, was her only reason for living. "Having my daughter was everything I ever wanted in life: one person in this world who loved me completely, totally, unconditionally. From the first time I looked into her eyes, that love, it was something I had never experienced. She loved me more than I loved myself. But it didn't heal me." After the loss of so many family members, Tracy's desire to die was even stronger, yet she refused to give in to those urges. "My daughter is very sensitive, very loving, and I knew that if I committed suicide, it would destroy her."

Never giving up, Tracy tried "various herbal remedies that helped to some extent, but it was never complete, probably because I didn't have the knowledge to prescribe for myself or stick with one thing long enough." Cost was also an issue.

"For many years I've been unable to hold steady employment, because when the depressions hit hard, I would lose work. The financial result was I've been living in poverty for most of my adult life." Unable to drive because of the drugs and panic attacks made finding work even more difficult. When she called me, Tracy and her daughter were living off government aid supplemented by charity from food pantries and shelters.

Her mental state was precarious. She broke into tears easily. "I don't think I go a few hours without sobbing. *Anything* can make me cry," she said. "At this point, I truly do not believe I will ever be well. My daughter is slipping away from me. Living alone with a mother who is this ill is having a terrible effect on her. I feel completely hopeless. I thought perhaps I could learn something from you."

Glimpses of Tracy's intelligence surfaced as we talked, and I sensed the internal struggle she was waging to hold herself together. She had physical challenges as well, obesity from years of psychiatric drugs and fibromyalgia that made walking painful. But Tracy was highly motivated and had done everything she could think of to help herself. Disability would pay for all the psychiatrists and psychiatric drugs in the world, but not for nondrug alternatives. She was trapped, with no resources or any family to help her.

I called Anne Procyk, a new naturopathic doctor who recently joined Natura Medica, the local group of holistic practitioners I personally used. She had spoken at one of my seminars, and I had been impressed by her quiet, thoughtful manner and knew she had some experience treating brain chemistry disorders. I explained Tracy's plight and asked if Anne would treat her at no charge if I could find someone to pay for the necessary supplements. She agreed. I called a friend who made a donation that covered the cost of Tracy's initial supplements.

On February 18, 2005, Tracy began working with Dr. Procyk. Tracy's treatment included two homeopathic medications (one in February and one in May), based on Tracy's detailed history, plus B-complex supplements, niacin, Pharmax fish oil, a women's vitamin/mineral/hormone formula, GABA, and additional supplements to treat her fibromyalgia. Tracy had nine appointments over the next seven months.

We talked as I drove Tracy to and from the appointments, but I never probed. Nor did I ever discuss her treatment directly with the doctor. It is critical that each person become responsible for her own healing. I listened, encouraging her when things were rocky and making suggestions of books to read or topics she might discuss with Dr. Procyk. As we talked following her appointment on August 30, Tracy was so much improved she hardly seemed like the same person.

I had no idea that the turnaround might be so fast because her symptoms had been severe and she had been on powerful, psychiatric drugs for so many years. Tracy was no longer constantly crying, talking about death, or groping to put a sentence together. Under Dr. Procyk's care, Tracy had stopped taking all psychiatric drugs when she started the natural regimen. Now she was usually smiling, talking lucidly. During our conversation she exclaimed, "It's *so great* to have my mind back!"

Tracy's interview for this chapter took place on September 28, 2005, seven months after she started holistic treatments. I asked if she could give me a month-by-month summary of the improvements she noticed.

When I met Anne, the wonderful initial thing was that this woman really cared. I'm not saying that medical doctors don't care, but this woman spent over an hour and a half talking to me. It wasn't like a psychotherapist who let me talk and said, "Uh-huh." This woman went through every tiny piece of my life. She probed the depths of how I was feeling, empathized with my pain, and obviously wanted to do anything she could to help me. She didn't dismiss things I would say that maybe sounded a little silly or far-fetched. Everything was very important in order for her to put together a program that would help me. I believed this woman would do whatever it took and not dismiss me after a couple of months if something wasn't working. I've experienced that a lot. Some doctors tend to get irritated when what they give you doesn't work.

What was my reaction to the first group of things she put me on? I went for weeks and didn't have a depressive episode. This was unbelievable to me. But she warned me this didn't mean I wouldn't have episodes, which eventually I did.

The first few months were a gentle roller coaster. What I noticed was it wasn't all highs and lows. I was getting even times, breaks of sunshine where just taking a walk with my dog could be a beautiful experience. My brain started working again. The gaps between my depressive episodes were longer, and I wasn't going right from a depressive episode into a manic episode. I was having "normal" time, something I hadn't experienced in twenty years.

I had tried working a couple of little jobs in the last few years, and nothing lasted more than two weeks. So I was feeling pretty shitty about myself. At the end of April, I applied for a job at a convenience store, absolutely terrified because I didn't think I could do it, with the register and computerized machines. My memory was so bad, I told my boss and coworkers that I would probably have to ask things more than once. I was fortunate to find a group [of people] who were very patient and helpful. When my paperwork didn't come out right, I couldn't figure out why because I still couldn't add and subtract properly. My assistant manager would figure it out for me, which was a blessing. Now, five months later, the paperwork is a breeze.

I love going to work. Sometimes it's hard to get going, get dressed, and walk to and from the store. But the minute I get there

and start working with people, especially after keeping myself se-
cluded for so long, it is such a joy.

At the very beginning when I had a few weeks of feeling so
much better, I started seeing humor. I'm witty again. I used to be
very funny, but I went through *years* where I never laughed. It's a
wonderful feeling to have somebody say something and come back
with a spontaneous comment.

The brightest ray of sunshine in all of this is that the change in
my daughter is unbelievable. When I was so sick, she ended up in
a group home two times. The state took her away from me, and I
fought very hard to get her back. She was withdrawn and angry,
acting out in destructive ways. Now, she has new friends who are
brighter, happier, and have goals. She has an amazing ability
with emotionally challenged children, and is working with them at
school. She's not worried about coming home and finding me
dead. She comes home and I'm cleaning the house, or I'm reading.
I'm not crying in bed—I'm *normal*.

I've just come from a M.D. who ran all kinds of physical tests
on me, and my entire health has improved. So, this isn't just feeding my brain, this is repairing all kinds of damage to my body. I
was hopeless and helpless and now I truly know you can come back
from this horrible disease.

The cost of Tracy's miraculous recovery over seven months was
$1,130 for Dr. Procyk's time (had she charged) and $1,155 for the natural supplements: $2,285 total. Anyone filling prescriptions knows this
is very inexpensive compared to the price of psychiatric drugs, but, of
course, the drugs are covered by insurance. Maintenance for Tracy
will run $2,000 a year, assuming $150 a month in supplements and two
naturopathic visits over twelve months. The cost is minuscule when
compared to years of government-funded pharmaceutical drug treatment, psychiatric therapy, hospital care, and disability payments.

As Tracy continues to restore her mind, her ability to work will improve, which will ultimately move her and her daughter out of

poverty. She is currently making plans to repair her old car, get her driver's license back, improve her job skills, and become an advocate of alternative mental health treatments for women and children living in poverty.

Your Steps to Health

Where do you start in trying to restore your mind? The first thing is this: *Do not discontinue or reduce your dose of psychiatric medications without the supervision of a physician.* Your brain has adjusted to the drugs you are taking, and any sudden changes may cause serious reactions and endanger your health.

Ask your doctor to help you find alternatives to prescription drugs. If your doctor is not receptive, find a new doctor who understands alternative treatments and will work with you. Under your doctor's supervision, begin supplying your body with vitamins, minerals, fish oils, and other vital elements needed for optimum health while eliminating substances that interfere with brain or central nervous system functions. As symptoms diminish, reduce the psychiatric medications you are taking, reporting to your doctor any serious mood or physical changes.

Each individual's biochemistry is unique. What works for one person may not work for you. What happens quickly for one may take longer for another. Recovering mental health is a process, not a quick fix, but it holds the promise of a cure instead of perpetual medication.

1. **Find a Special Doctor.** When I was trying to heal myself four years ago, no primary care doctor or psychiatrist I spoke with believed in alternative treatments for bipolar disorder or would even meet with me to discuss them. With all the bad press about drug side effects since then, that is changing. However, finding a doctor to guide you can be tricky. Conventionally trained medical doctors and psychiatrists are only

taught to heal mental disorders with drugs, and few will acknowledge that other treatments exist. Naturopathic and orthomolecular physicians (medical doctors who rely mainly on nutrients instead of drugs) are trained to use alternatives to heal all types of diseases, but they may not know how to treat bipolar disorder with alternatives, especially if they were schooled ten or more years ago. I recommend naturopaths because they are more common and have specialized training in eliminating the underlying causes of all disease, healing totally without drugs with more experience using natural substances. Naturopaths are also relatively inexpensive, charging $75–$150 a visit, which is covered by a few enlightened insurance companies in certain states.

If you hear of a wonderful M.D. who uses alternatives extensively, however, then go to her or him. My point is this: There are no perfect doctors for this process. In all professions, there are a few who are exceptional. Pick the best practitioner you can find with a track record of success using alternative therapies, one who treats you with respect, and whom you like. Work with him three to six months and see if you experience obvious improvements. If not, change doctors.

See, the resources section for Web sites and telephone referral networks to assist in locating alternative practitioners near you. Another method I use is to ask a variety of people within the alternative healing industry (massage therapists, acupuncturists, owners of health food stores, and the like) which naturopathic doctor has the best reputation for results in the community. If you hear the same name from several different sources, make an appointment to talk with that doctor.

Because the American diet is so unhealthy, any doctor using alternatives will recommend dramatic dietary changes to nourish your brain and eliminate substances that interfere with central nervous system functions. Follow them. Not everyone can afford organic foods, but many people find that their budget goes a lot further when they are no longer buying expensive packaged, processed, and energy-draining junk foods and sodas.

2. **Take the Basics.** Begin taking high-quality vitamin/mineral supplements, fish oils, and perhaps amino acids.

> **Vitamins/Minerals.** Buy high-potency blends and the best quality you can afford. Look specifically for blends that include at least 50 mg of most B-vitamins, 200 mcg of selenium, 200 mcg of chromium, and small amounts of biotin. If you can afford the combination blends that have vitamins/minerals/amino acids all in one (see resources), they may be less expensive than buying these substances separately.

> **Fish Oils.** Since most Americans are deficient in omega-3 fatty acids, you'll need to take more at first: 3 to 5 grams (3,000–5,000 mg) daily, depending on body size. (They do thin the blood slightly, so if you are on prescription blood thinners, do not take them without first consulting your doctor.)

> Fish oils are unstable, so the best ones will be kept refrigerated (you should store them there too) and contain small amounts of vitamin E to help maintain their quality. Be sure the brand is filtered, free of heavy metals and other toxins found in all fish today. I used Dr. Andrew Stoll's Omega Brite brand initially because it is formulated to contain seven times more EPA than DHA than other brands, and his studies showed that EPA was the mood-lifting element. However, natural fish oils contain a different balance, a 1.5:1 ratio of EPA to DHA.

> After two years, I switched to a brand containing the natural ratio, which was also less expensive. I currently use

Pharmax, an orange-flavored liquid fish oil that tastes fine and reduces the number of capsules I take every day. Other good brands are Nature's Bounty and Nordic Naturals (this also comes in small, flavored chewables designed for children). Although flaxseed oil is an omega-3 fat, it has a different composition than fish oil and has not been tested on people with psychiatric illnesses. Cod liver oil should be avoided, because, according to Dr. Stoll, at the high doses needed for therapeutic use, it will deliver toxic amounts of vitamin A.[1]

Amino Acids. I did not use amino acid supplements initially, but several others in this book found them very helpful. To alter mood, always take amino acids between meals (not with food)—before breakfast, in the late afternoon, or at bedtime. Discuss the following with your doctor:

Tryptophan (sold as 5-HTP), 50–150 mg, for depression, stress, and to curb carbohydrate cravings.

Tyrosine or **Phenylalanine** (or a combo, since tyrosine is made from phenylalanine), 500 mg, two or three times a day (too much can trigger mania), to lift depression, aid in stress management, promote memory, and suppress appetite.

GABA, 500 mg, as needed, to calm down or for sleep (sometimes blended with taurine and glycine for calming).

Glutamine, 1,000 mg three times a day, to make more GABA and promote intelligence or memory while healing leaky gut and reducing alcohol or sugar cravings.

Methionine, 500 mg, twice a day to lower blood histamine, which, when elevated, contributes to mania and anxiety.

Cysteine and **Cystine, Methionine,** and **Glutamic Acid**—all sulfur-containing amino acids that aid in detoxification.

Taurine, Methionine, and **Glutamine** to improve fat digestion and absorption of fat-soluble vitamins.

Balanced Amino Acids. If you are a vegan, vegetarian, or do not like or digest protein well, try taking a balanced amino acid formulation. I like Platinum Plus, developed by a holistic chiropractor, Dr. Brice Vickery, and now sold by Life Enthusiast Co-op (www.life-enthusiast.com).

3. **Rule Out Underlying Causes.** Have a complete physical, asking your doctor to review all your prescriptions and illnesses for mood disorder side effects. Order the following tests, using the knowledge of your history and symptoms to guess which causes are most likely, testing them first:

A blood panel for vitamin/mineral deficiencies

Thyroid and adrenal panels (also check for Wilson's thyroid syndrome)

Blood and hair analysis for heavy metals (toxic chemicals, if suspected)

Pyroluria, methlyation, and other inborn errors of metabolism

Hormone testing for men and women (using only *natural* hormone supplements!)

Urinary peptide tests for gluten and casein sensitivity

IgA, IgE blood tests for food allergies/sensitivities

Stool samples for candida yeast, bacteria, and parasites

4. **Options from Part II.** If you, or a minor with depression or bipolar disorder under your care, are a personality that tends not to follow doctor's recommendations, and most likely won't take supplements or follow dietary restrictions faithfully, find a homeopathic practitioner to prescribe a liquid medication that you simply take twice daily. Minors may also enjoy learning to retrain their brain waves with neurofeedback, since it uses a computer feedback system. Or consider therapeutic touch or another energy-balancing modality to resolve the illness energetically, which in time can reduce the physical symptoms. If you have suffered abuse or trauma, find a psychotherapist and do EMDR therapy in conjunction with treatment by a physician.

5. **Withdrawal from Psychiatric Drugs.** Most doctors recommend very gradually reducing the psychiatric drug dose over time. As you have read in these chapters, however, people often go off medications cold turkey and, if taking the high-potency supplements, may not have withdrawal symptoms. Alternative clinics try to get patients off psychiatric medications as soon as possible because the drugs can actually cause the very symptoms they are supposed to cure.

Withdrawal side effects vary depending on how long it takes for a drug to wash out of your system. Since Prozac takes weeks, it has fewer withdrawal symptoms. Paxil and Luvox wash out in just a couple of days, causing reactions in 50 percent and 86 percent of patients, respectively.[2] Each psychiatric drug will be different. Because withdrawal symptoms often resemble those of the illness, it can be difficult to figure out the source of your symptoms.

Common Antidepressant Withdrawal Effects

Anxiety, agitation (commonly mistaken for returning symptoms of the disorder)

Crying spells, irritability

Loss of equilibrium: dizziness, spinning sensations, difficulty walking

Gastrointestinal symptoms: nausea, vomiting

Flulike symptoms: fatigue, lethargy, muscle pain, chills

Sensory disturbances: tingling, electric-shock sensations

Sleep disturbances: insomnia, vivid dreams

Disorientation, confusion, memory problems

Source: J. Glen Mullen, M.D., *Prozac Backlash* (New York: Simon & Schuster, 2000), 72.

6. Persist! Seldom does one doctor have all the answers, nor do they have time to give detailed explanations about why you should do what they recommend. Work with a doctor for several months, provided you see steady improvement. Alternative therapies take time because the natural substances used in these approaches gradually help repair and rebuild the body's own systems. However, you should notice subtle improvements within a month or two, significant changes within six months, and a gradual restoration of mental health within a year or two.

The process I advocate does not guarantee an easy cure for your depression or bipolar disorder. There are far too many variables. Like cancer, mental illness has confounded years of research because it is multicausal. Successful recovery depends as much on your commitment and efforts as the skills of practitioners guiding you.

This book presents many of the most likely underlying causes of depression or bipolar symptoms, real-life examples to demonstrate that healing is possible, and a basic outline of how each treatment spurs healing. My hope is that I have given you enough information—and the promise of success—for you to try healing depression or bipolar disorder without drugs.

Anti-Inflammatory Diet

Specific foods cause the body to create excessive arachidonic acid, which results in inflammation. This, in turn, contributes to Alzheimer's disease, arthritis, tumor growth, and many other illnesses. This diet, provided by my naturopath at Natura Medica, lowers the production of arachidonic acid.

AVOID	DO EAT (ORGANIC WHEN POSSIBLE)
Red meat	Chicken, Turkey ("free range," antibiotic & hormone free)
Fried foods, saturated fats, trans fats/hydrogenated oils	
Sugar, artificial sweeteners	Fish (limited to 1–2 times a week due to mercury and pollutants and avoiding raw shellfish)
Refined foods, flours & white rice	
Dairy products	Legumes, such as peas, beans, lentils
Wheat products, such as pasta, breads, cereals	Whole grains, except wheat

AVOID	DO EAT (ORGANIC WHEN POSSIBLE)
Peanuts or peanut oil	Soy products, such as tofu, tempeh, soy cheese
Soft drinks, sweetened juices	Eggs, organic and hormone-free *only*
Coffee, black tea, colas, & chocolate	4–5 vegetables a day, 2 raw
Alcohol	2–3 fruits a day of differing colors
Hormones; exposure to herbicides or pesticides	Nuts and seeds
	Essential fatty acids, omega-3s, -6s, and -9s
	Small quantities of "good" oils, such as olive, canola, walnut—none highly heated by frying
	Filtered water, herbal teas, green tea, vegetable juices, diluted unsweetened fruit juices

Tips:

- Eat 4–8 ounces of protein per day, not per meal. Protein is the primary fuel for cellular replacement and repair, but too much protein in the diet contributes to osteoporosis.

- To test your *sensitivity* to any suspected food, stop eating it for three weeks, then enjoy it three times in one day. Monitor how you feel over the subsequent forty-eight hours, watching for fatigue, stiffness, headaches, and the like. Obviously, *do not* do this with foods you know you are *allergic* to.

- Carbohydrates give sustained energy, yet people's needs and metabolism vary widely. By eliminating wheat, you'll cut back and probably drop pounds, but do eat some whole grains or you'll feel hungry all the time. When you're hungry, eat something nutritious, avoiding empty calories. Do not snack more than once every two or three hours, because each time you put something in your mouth (even a tiny candy), the body releases insulin, the "hunger hormone." Constant snacking will actually increase your hunger, while three small meals and two healthy snacks a day will keep your blood sugar, mood, and energy levels steady.

Sample Candida Control Program by Infinity Health*

Length of Program: Four Months

Important Note:
Before embarking on this Candida Control Program, be sure to rule out the presence of parasites. When parasites are present, the Candida Program is often not fully successful. If you're unsure of the presence of parasites, consider one of the following: (1) Do laboratory testing for parasites, or (2) Take the DE-P Formula (in appendix C) as a trial (two to three capsules twice daily on an empty stomach) for one month. If significant improvement is noted, this may suggest the benefit of doing additional laboratory testing to identify parasites, or starting preferred treatment (see Anti-Protozoa Program, appendix C).

This program includes the following elements:

Combat Fung: A natural antifungal, antiyeast and anticandida fighter. Combat Fung capsules have been the cornerstone of

---

* Many thanks to Timothy Kuss, M.A., C.N.C., for permitting inclusion of this protocol. For further information, please contact Infinity Health in Littleton, Colorado, at (800) 733–9293 or (303) 703–3772.

Infinity Health's highly successful anticandida program for many years. Powerful and effective, yet well tolerated. (See note on next page.)

Biotin: Often overlooked, biotin is an important member of the B-vitamin family. It is necessary for carbohydrate, fat, and protein metabolism, and aids in the utilization of other B-vitamins. It is vital to the health of the skin and intestinal tract. Signs of deficiency include muscle pain, poor appetite, depression, and yeast/candida overgrowth.

Oregano Oil: Oregano oil contains two antioxidant phenolic compounds—thymol and carvacrol. Research shows they have antiyeast, anticandida, as well as broad antimicrobial properties. This product is a mainstay in many candida and parasite control programs.

Grapeseed Extract: Superior antioxidant protection. Contains flavonoid compounds (minimum 90 percent total polyphenols), which have 20–50 times more antioxidant activity than vitamins C and E. Grapeseed extract is a more potent free- radical scavenger for two reasons: (1) It neutralizes *both* water- and fat-soluble free radicals, and (2) it acts within the cell membrane to preserve living tissue. It is especially protective of blood vessel linings and targets LDL cholesterol.

Garlic (Pure-Gar™): High-potency, odorless garlic tablets. Pure-Gar® garlic is processed by a proprietary quick cool/dry method that maintains certified minimum levels of alliin, allicin yield, total thiosulfanates, gamma glutamyl cysteines, and total sulfur compounds. The therapeutic value of whole fresh garlic is retained, yet its pungent odor is masked by the tablet's enteric coating.

NutriBiotic GSE®: General antimicrobial tablets with certified organic grapefruit extract used in antiyeast, anticandida, antibacteria, and antiprotoza programs.

A.D.P: Softgels containing two antioxidant phenolic compounds, thymol and carvacrol, with broad antimicrobial properties.

A-F (F-GAL): Used for centuries in the tropical rain forest as herbal medicine to treat fungi and yeast. Clinical documentation confirms many of the botanicals in A-F capsules possess in vitro and and/or in vivo properties. (See note below.)

Multi-Flora ABF: A full-spectrum probiotic to help restore friendly flora to the intestinal tract. Combines two friendly, compatible microorganisms in capsule form: *Lactobacillus acidophilus* (DDS strain) and *Bifidus longum*, in a FOS and rice starch base.

Note: If coffee is consumed in the morning, take Combat Fung or A-F at midmorning or midafternoon, away from food and coffee.

Month 1

WEEK 1

Upon Arising: Take 1 capsule Combat Fung (away from food and coffee).

With Breakfast: 1 capsule biotin (1,000 mcg) and 1 capsule oregano oil or A.D.P and 1 NutriBiotic GSE tablet.

With Lunch & Dinner: 1 capsule oregano oil or A.D.P and 1 NutriBiotic GSE tablet.

WEEKS 2–4

Upon Arising: Take 1 capsule Combat Fung (away from food and coffee).

With Breakfast: 1 capsule biotin (1,000 mcg) and 1 capsule oregano oil or A.D.P and 1 NutriBiotic GSE tablet.

With Lunch & Dinner: 1 capsule oregano oil or A.D.P and 1 NutriBiotic GSE tablet.

Bedtime: Take 1 capsule Combat Fung (away from food). Take with a large glass of water.

Month 2

Upon Arising: Take 2 A-F capsules (away from food and coffee).

With Breakfast: 1 capsule biotin (1,000 mcg) and 1 tablet Pure-Gar and 1 NutriBiotic GSE tablet.

With Lunch & Dinner: 1 tablet Pure-Gar and 1 NutriBiotic GSE tablet.

Bedtime: Take 2 capsules A-F (away from food). Take with a large glass of water.

Month 3

Upon Arising: Take 2 capsules of Multi-Flora.

15–30 Minutes Later: Take 1 capsule Combat Fung (away from food and coffee).

With Breakfast: 1 capsule biotin (1,000 mcg) and 1 capsule oregano oil or A.D.P and 1 NutriBiotic GSE tablet.

With Lunch & Dinner: 1 capsule oregano oil or A.D.P and 1 NutriBiotic GSE tablet.

Bedtime: Take 1 capsule Combat Fung (away from food). Take with a large glass of water.

Month 4

Upon Arising: Continue taking 2 capsules of the Multi-Flora until bottle is finished.

With Meals: Finish bottles of oregano oil or A.D.P and NutriBiotic GSE by taking 1 each with all meals.

Throughout the entire program: Eat moderately. Eat plenty of fresh vegetables, especially steamed or lightly sautéed in the beginning. Increase the raw vegetables slowly over the course of the four months. Eat moderate servings of protein, such as fish, meat, tofu, nuts and seeds, and beans, if tolerated. Vegetable oils such as olive, grapeseed, flaxseed, and sesame are recommended. Eat sparingly from the grain group (one to two *small* servings daily). Best choices are basmati, corn, and quinoa. Of course, avoid sugar and sweets (including cookies, muffins, pancakes, ice cream, etc.), as well as alcohol, wheat, milk, and cheese. Avoid fruit juice, oranges, melons, bananas, and dried fruits. Neutral fruits, such as apples, kiwi, berries, plums, apricots, and pears are usually okay in moderation (one to two pieces daily). Some individuals may have to restrict these fruits completely for a time.

Professional Notes

1. Patients with a chronically weak immune system are advised to take one of the following as well: Systemic's Gt (Thymus) or LFI's Master Defense. Both are excellent for enhancing and strengthening the overall immune response.
2. Drink plenty of fluids, especially purified water and teas, such as ginger, pau d'arco, hyssop, spearmint, or raspberry. A ginger and pau d'arco blend is particularly tasty, as well as therapeutic.
3. Highly sensitive and/or reactive patients need to ease into this program very slowly. Refer to the instructions on the Combat Fung bottle for Very Sensitive Types. Follow the same procedure when A-F is started. This minimizes and usually avoids die-off (Herxheimer) reactions.
4. For tougher cases, consider taking Systemic's #4 Fungdx.
5. If taking a multiple vitamin high in biotin (such as True Balance or Glucobalance), additional biotin is *not* needed at breakfast.

Sample Antiprotozoa Program by Infinity Health*

Length of Program: Ten to Fourteen Weeks

Protozoa infections have become increasingly prevalent in recent years, in the United States as well as overseas. Protozoa are opportunistic, potentially pathogenic, single-celled organisms that can take up residence in the gastrointestinal tract of humans as well as in pets or other animals. This botanical-based program has been tested with hundreds of patients over the past few years. It has proven itself successful in a majority of cases. It is designed to be effective against the following protozoa: *Blastocystis hominis, Cryptosporidium parvum, Dientamoeba fragilis, Endolimax nana, Entamoeba coli, Entamoeba hartmanni*, and *Giardia lamblia*.

This program is based on two separate one-week cycles, alternated every other week for a total of ten weeks. **Note:** *Blastocystis hominis* or chronic protozoa infections usually take an additional four weeks, for a total of fourteen weeks, rather than the normal ten. In certain mild cases, an individual may require fewer than ten weeks. In other exceptional cases, more than fourteen weeks may be necessary.

---

* Many thanks to Timothy Kuss, M.A., C.N.C., for permitting inclusion of this protocol. For further information, please contact Infinity Health in Littleton, Colorado, at (800) 733–9293 or (303) 703–3772.

The program consists of the following elements:

Black Walnut/Wormwood Herbal Complex: Combines a variety of powerful antiparasitic botanicals in liquid extract form.

ATAK (Immune Rejuvenator): A powerful formula, from Systemic Formulas, which helps to ferret out the presence of deep-seated and/or stubborn protozoal infections.

DE-P Formula: A classical blend of potent antiparasitic herbs in capsule form from a master herbalist at Osage Natural Health Center. Also has antiyeast, anticandida benefits.

NutriBiotic GSE® (Grapefruit Seed Extract): A broad-spectrum, antimicrobial formula.

Oregano Oil: Gelcaps possess generalized antimicrobial properties.

A-P: A powerful antiparasite formula from the rain forests of Brazil, where parasitic infection is quite common. A-P has been used successfully for many years.

WO (Wonder Oil): A potent, aromatic blend of antimicrobial extracts, including Worm Seed (Artemesia) and Leptotaenia oils. Highly concentrated; use *only* 1–3 drops.

VRM3 (Micro Pathogens): An antiprotozoa botanical mixture from Systemic Formulas, which relies on a unique blend of North and South American herbs.

Optional Additional Formulas

Clove Capsules: Fresh clove caps have strong antimicrobial and antiparasitic properties, especially helpful in killing the eggs of larger parasites.

Gastromycin with Bismuth: In capsule form from Allergy Research. Has lumen-active antimicrobial and antiprotozoa activity.

MSM (Methylsulfonylmethane): Used in veterinary medicine for years as an effective antiparasitic agent. A rich source of organic sulfur (parasites do *not* like sulfur) with general anti-inflammatory properties.

Paracidin: A fatty acid complex with molecular iodine absorbed to activated charcoal.

Accel: A comprehensive nutritional beverage powder containing over 100 different vitamins, minerals, amino acids, and herbs that support key body systems.

Seacure: Deep ocean whitefish especially processed to utilize peptide chain amino acids. Capsules help rebuild, restore, and heal the GI tract.

Cycle 1 (Weeks 1, 3, 5, 7, 9)

Upon Arising and at Bedtime: 2 A-P, 2 VRM3, 1 ATAK with 2–3 drops of WO in an empty capsule.

With all 3 Meals: 1 oregano oil capsule.

Cycle 2 (Weeks 2, 4, 6, 8, 10)

Upon Arising and at Bedtime: 3 DE-P, 1 ATAK, 1 dropper Black Walnut/Wormwood Complex (15–18 drops) with 2–3 drops of WO in an empty capsule.

With All 3 Meals: 1 NutriBiotic GSE tablet.

Professional Notes

1. Individuals who are sensitive and/or reactive to various botanical supplements should take 1 capsule of ACX (Detoxifier) 2–3 times daily. Formula ACX reduces toxicity in the bloodstream, supports liver and kidney functions, and helps to avoid healing crises/reactions.
2. During this program, it is especially important to maintain daily bowel functions. If constipation should occur, take extra magnesium or a vegetable-based fiber product, such as Fiber Greens (Orange Peel) or Smooth Food 2 (New Chapter), or a gentle herbal laxative product, such as Formula C (Colon) or AO (Aloe Vera) from Systemic Formulas.
3. Protozoa infections may be spread from one family member to another. It is best to test all family members via stool analysis to be certain. Sexual partners should be treated simultaneously to reduce the risk of reinfection to each other.
4. Beware of potential sources of reinfection, including unwashed or inadequately washed fruits and vegetables, contaminated water, pets, and gardening with bare hands and feet. Leo Galland, M.D., has warned against eating at salad bars for this reason.
5. Our first lines of defense against parasites include a healthy immune system and a competent digestive tract. When gastric

and digestive juices are sufficient, parasites, including protozoa, are destroyed in the highly acidic environment of the
stomach. If a patient has insufficient hydrochloric acid output, parasites can gain a foothold in the body. Digestive enzyme supplementation is appropriate in these cases.

6. After completing the above program, it is best to wait at least
2 weeks *before* retesting via a second stool analysis. It is ideal
to complete 1 month of the bowel recolonization program
(see below) before retesting.

7. The above program is effective in approximately 80–85 percent of cases. With more difficult patients, the addition of a
tissue-active antiamoebicidal drug, such as Tinidazol
(Fazigyn), may be appropriate. This medication needs to be
prescribed by a physician. Prescriptions can be filled by
Cronos Pharmacy in Las Vegas, Nevada, (800) 723–7455.

Bowel Recolonization & Healing Program: For One Month Immediately Following the Antiprotozoa Program

After completion of the antiprotozoa program, it is important to
reestablish the health and integrity of the intestinal tract. The recolonization of the healthy, beneficial flora, and healing of the sensitive
small intestine villi and microvilli, are crucial for this purpose. The
following formulas are designed to strengthen and rebuild the intestinal tract and enhance optimal absorption of nutrients.

Upon Arising and at Bedtime (away from food):
2 Multi-Flora ABF capsules (UAS Laboratories) *or* 2 ABC capsules (Systemic Formulas)
1 teaspoon AO (concentrated Aloe Vera—Systemic Formulas)
2 L-glutamine (500 mg)

Once or Twice Daily

2-1 scoop (included) Accel powder (nutritional beverage mix) in water or juice

With Food

2 Seacure capsules 3 times per day

Optional: Helpful Formula to Maximize Intestinal Rebuilding

2 DSIR (Digestant/Internal Regenerator—Systemic Formulas)

Resources:
Natural Alternatives for Healing

Referral Organizations

American Association of Naturopathic Physicians
4435 Wisconsin Avenue, NW, Suite 403
Washington, DC 20026
(202) 237–8150
(866) 538–2267 toll free
www.naturopathic.org with search/referral system

In addition to basic medical sciences and conventional diagnosis, naturopathic physicians (N.D.s) are the highest trained practitioners in the broad scope of alternative medicine. This includes therapeutic nutrition, botanical medicine, homeopathy, natural childbirth, classical Chinese medicine, hydrotherapy, naturopathic manipulative therapy, pharmacology, and minor surgery.

American College for Advancement in Medicine (ACAM)
23121 Verdugo Drive, Suite 204
Laguna Hills, CA 92653
(949) 583–7666
(800) 532–3688 toll free
www.acam.org with search/referral system

ACAM is the largest and oldest nonprofit medical society dedicated to educating physicians and other health care professionals on the latest findings and emerging procedures in preventive/nutritional (alternative) medicine.

EEG Institute
22020 Clarendon Street, #305
Woodland Hills, CA 91367
(818) 373–1334
www.eeginfo.com with search/referral system

The EEG Institute is the clinic and research center of the Brian Othmer Foundation, a nonprofit dedicated to research, education, and clinical services in neurofeedback.

National Center for Homeopathy
801 North Fairfax Street, Suite 306
Alexandria, VA 22314
(703) 548–7790
www.homeopathic.org with search/referral system

NCH is the leading open-membership organization supporting and promoting homeopathy in the U.S.

Safe Harbor
787 West Woodbury Road, #2
Altadena, CA 91001
(626) 791–7868
www.alternativementalhealth.com with search/referral system

A nonprofit educating the public, medical practitioners, and the government about safe alternative mental health treatments. Seminars meet the requirements of the Accreditation Council for Continuing Medical Education.

Well Mind Association of Greater Washington
P.O. Box 201
Kensington, MD 20895
(301) 774–6617

Well Mind Association of Greater Washington is a nonprofit clearinghouse for alternative mental health information and referrals.

Practitioners or Clinics Appearing in This Book

Victoria L. Ibric, M.D., Ph.D. (neurofeedback)
Neurofeedback/NeuroRehab Institute
65 North Madison Avenue, #405
Pasadena, CA 91101
(626) 577–2202
www.neurofeedback-dribric.com

Stephen Leighton, M.D.
Family Care Health & Wellness Center (medical wellness center)
1430 HSA Lane
Winston-Salem, NC 27101
(336) 723–9002

Andrew Levinson, M.D. (orthomolecular internist and psychiatrist)
Vitality Health & Wellness
2999 NE 191st Street, #905
Aventura, FL 33180
(305) 466–1100
www.vitalitywellness.com

Henry Mann, M.D. (psychiatry and neurofeedback)
188 Wolf Neck Road
Stonington, CT 06378
(860) 536–6023

Neecie Moore, Ph.D. (psychotherapy & glyconutrients)
Life Coaching Institute
4009 Old Denton Road
Carrollton, TX 75007
(214) 739–6644

Deirdre J. O'Connor, N.D., and Anne Procyk, N.D.
Natura Medica (alternative wellness clinic)
12 Roosevelt Avenue
Mystic, CT 06355
(860) 572–9566

Pfeiffer Treatment Center & Health Research Institute (clinic & brain research center)
4575 Weaver Parkway
Warrenville, IL 60555
(630) 505–0300
www.hriptc.org

Julia Ross, M.A.
Recovery Systems (mood, addiction, & eating disorders)
147 Lomita Drive, Suite D
Mill Valley, CA 94941
(415) 383–3611 ext #1
www.moodcure.com

Tim Shannon, N.D. (classical homeopathy)
2610 SE Clinton Street, Suite E
Portland, OR 97202
(503) 236–8853
www.drtshannon.com

Other Practitioners Who Treat Mood Disorders Without Drugs (listed by state)

John Dommisse, M.D., Tucson, AZ (520) 577–1940,
    www.johndommisseemd.com
Clark Hansen, N.D. (children's homeopathy), Scotsdale, AZ (480) 991–5092

Dorothea Cist, N.D., Brain Therapeutics Medical Clinic (& reversing brain injury), Mission Viejo, CA (949) 367–8870, www.strokedoctor.com

Robert Cathcart, M.D., Los Altos, CA (650) 949–2822, www.orthomed.com

Paul Berger, M.D., Boulder, CO (303) 449–3100

James Gordon, M.D., Center for Mind–Body Medicine, Washington, DC (202) 537–6837, www.cmbm.org

Linda Rayner, M.D., Atlanta, GA (770) 390–0012

Alan Bain, D.O., Chicago, IL (312) 236–7010, www.cihi.net

Myrna Trowbridge, D.O., D.C., Valparaiso, IN (219) 462–3377

George Wolverton, M.D., Clarksville, IN (812) 282–4309

Ronald Hunninghake, M.D., Center for the Improvement of Human Functioning, Wichita, KS (316) 682–3100, www.brightspot.org

Laue Shaffia, M.D. (environmental medicine & homeopathy) Lawrence, KS (785) 841–1243

Robert Novak, D.C./C.C.N., Kansas City, KS (913) 788–7300

Stephen Kiteck, M.D., Somerset, KY (606) 677–0459

James Odell, M.D., Louisville, KY (502) 429–8835, biologicalmedicine. info

Stephanie F. Cave, M.D. (author, *What Your Doctor May Not Tell You About Children's Vaccinations*), Baton Rouge, LA (225) 767–7433

Mark D. Mincolla, Ph.D. (nutrition), Cohasset, MA (781) 383–6554, www.maxhealing.com

Barry Taylor, N.D., New England Family Health Center, Weston, MA (781) 237–8505, www.drbarrytaylor.com

Alice Lee-Bloem, M.D. (orthomolecular psychiatry), Olney, MD (301) 802–4474

Alan Weiner, D.O., Portland, ME (207) 828–8080

Devra Krassner, N.D., Portland, ME (207) 828–8080

Nedra Downing, D.O., Clarkston, MI (248) 625–6677

Health Recovery Center (& addictions), Minneapolis, MN (612) 827–7800 or (800) 554–9155, www.healthrecovery.com

Laurie Allen, D.C., L.A.C. (and nutrition), Poplar Bluff, MO 573 778–0500, www.allenwellnesscenter.com

Tipu Sulton, M.D., Florissant, MO (314) 921–5600

Margaret Beeson, N.D., Billings, MT (406) 259–5096

Jameson Starbuck, N.D., Missoula, MT (406) 549–0005

Mark Eisen, M.D. (& homeopathy), Chapel Hill, NC (919) 967–9452

Richard Ash, M.D., New York, NY (212) 758–3200
Eric Braverman, M.D., Path Medical Clinic, New York, NY (212) 213–6155
Michael B. Schachter, M.D./C.N.S., Schachter Center for Complementary
    Medicine, Suffern, NY (845) 368–4700, www.schachtercenter.com
Joseph Wojcik, M.D., Bronxville, NY (914) 793–6161
Bonnie Camo, M.D. (nutrition & homeopathy), Kendall Park, NJ (732)
    422–1585
Mary Alice Cooper, M.D. (& homeopathy), Albuquerque, NM (505)
    266–6522
Steven W. Weiss, M.D., Albuquerque, NM (505) 872–2611
Terry Chappell, M.D., Bluffton, OH (419) 358–4627
Janet McNiel, M.D., Knoxville, TN (865) 525–2121
John Parks Trowbridge, M.D., Humble, TX (281) 540–2329
Dennis Remington, M.D., Provo, UT (801) 373–8500
Bruce Semon, M.D., Ph.D., Milwaukee, WI (414) 962–6100

Canadian Practitioners

Abraham Hoffer, M.D. (leading orthomolecular pioneer, now retired but
    willing to consult with physicians), Victoria, British Columbia, Canada
    (250) 386–8756
Jennifer Armstrong, M.D., Nepean, Ontario, Canada (613) 721–9800

Combination Vitamin/Mineral/Amino Acid Supplements

EMPowerplus, www.truehope.com, (888) 878–3467
Equilib, www.equilib.us, (866) 437–7093
Quiet Minds, www.quietminds.us, (877) 601–7363

Glyconutrients

Mannatech, www.mannatech.com, (800) 281–4469

Fish Oil Supplements

Omega Brite, www.omegabrite.com, (800) 383–2030 or (888) 456–6342
Pharmax Finest Fish Oil, www.pharmaxllc.com (sell only through health
    care practitioners, not direct to consumers)
Nordic Naturals, www.nordicnaturals.com, (800) 662–2544
Nature's Bounty, www.naturesbounty.com, (800) 433–2990

Allergy/Candida/Parasite Testing Laboratory

Great Smokies Diagnostic Laboratory
63 Zillicoa Street
Asheville, NC 28801
www.gsdl.com
(828) 285–2223

Pyroluria Testing Laboratory

Bio Center Laboratory
3100 North Hillside
Wichita, KS 67219
(800) 494–7785

Compounding Pharmacy for Thyroid T_3

Mountain View Pharmacy
10565 North Tatum Boulevard, #B-118
Paradise Valley, AZ 85253
(480) 948–7065 or (800) 942–7065

Nonchemical Gardening and Cleaning

Earth Friendly Alternatives to herbicides, pesticides, and household chemicals (award-winning, 62-page booklet, published by the Stonington [CT] Garden Club), www.stonington-gardenclub.org.

Informative Web Sites

www.alternativementalhealth.com: Scientific articles, testimonials, and information on healing all mental disorders without drugs

www.truehope.com: Bipolar supplements and information

www.brodabarnes.org: Thyroid & metabolic balance

www.wilsonsthyroidsyndrome.com: Subclinical thyroid condition (doctor's free tech support telephone 800-420-5801)

www.emdr.com: Eye Movement Desensitization & Reprocessing (EMDR)

www.eegsupport.com: Neurofeedback

www.homeopathic.org: National Center for Homeopathy

www.loomisenzymes.com: Natural enzyme supplements

Recommended Reading

Weintraub, Skye, N.D., *Allergies and Holistic Healing*. Pleasant Grove, UT: Woodland Publishing, 1997.

Lesser, Michael, M.D., *The Brain Chemistry Diet*. New York: Penguin Putnam, 2002.

Khalsa, Dharma Singh, M.D., *Brain Longevity*. New York: Warner Books, 1997.

Elkins, Rita, *Depression and Natural Medicine*. Pleasant Grove, UT: Woodland Publishing, 1995.

Cousens, Gabriel, M.D., *Depression-Free for Life*. New York: HarperCollins, 2000.

Baker, Sidney M., M.D., *Detoxification and Healing*. New York: McGraw-Hill, 2004.

DeFelice, Karen, *Enzymes for Autism and other Neurological Conditions*. Thundersnow Interactive: 2003. defelice@thunde4rsnow.com

Brennan, Barbara, *Hands of Light: A Guide to Healing Through the Human Energy Field*. New York: Bantam Doubleday Dell Publishing, 1988.

Lansky, Amy, Ph.D., *Impossible Cure: the Promise of Homeopathy*. R. L. Ranch Press: 2003. Portola Valley, CA. www.impossiblecure.com

Ross, Julia, M.A., *The Mood Cure*. New York: Penguin Books, 2002.

Marohn, Stephanie, *The Natural Medicine Guide to Bipolar Disorder*. Charlottesville, VA: Hampton Roads Publishing, 2003.

Kirschmann, Gayla J., and John D. Kirschmann, *Nutrition Almanac*. New York: McGraw-Hill, 1996.

Stoll, Andrew L., M.D., *The Omega–3 Connection*. New York: Simon & Schuster, 2001.

Glenmullen, Joseph, M.D., *Prozac Backlash*. New York: Simon & Schuster, 2000.

Gerber, Richard, M.D., *Vibrational Medicine*. Rochester, VT: Bear & Company, 2001.

Weintraub, Amy, *Yoga for Depression*. New York: Random House, 2004.

Breggin, Peter R., M.D., and David Cohen, Ph.D., *Your Drug May Be Your Problem*. New York: HarperCollins, 1999.

Notes

Introduction

1. National Institute of Mental Health summary of mental disorder statistics, 2006, reported at www.nimh.nih.gov/publicat/numbers.cfm.
2. National Center for Health Statistics figures reported by the American Association of Suicidology at www.suicidology.org.
3. National Institute of Mental Health summary of mental disorder statistics, 2006, reported at www.nimh.nih.gov/publicat/numbers.cfm.
4. K. R. Jamison, M.D., "Suicide and Bipolar Disorder," *Journal of Clinical Psychiatry* 61, Supplement, no. 9 (2000): 47–51.
5. www.alternativementalhealth.com.
6. J. Biederman, et al., "Attention-Deficit Hyperactivity Disorder and Juvenile Mania; an Overlooked Comorbidity," *Journal of the American Academy of Child and Adolescent Psychiatry* 35 (1996): 997–1008.
7. *American College of Physicians Complete Home Medical Guide* (New York: DK Publishing, 1999), 512.
8. *Principles of Neural Science* (New York: Elsevier Science, 1991), 24–26.
9. Bill Buxton, "Forward into the Past," *Time* (October 11, 2004): 80.
10. *Treatment of Depression—Newer Pharmacotherapies, Summary, Evidence Report/Technology Assessment* no. 7, March 1999 (Rockville, MD: Agency for Health Care Policy and Research, 1999).
11. J. Glenmullen, M.D., *Prozac Backlash* (New York: Simon & Schuster, 2000), 190.
12. M. Angell, M.D., *The Truth About the Drug Companies: How They Deceive Us and What to Do About It* (New York: Random House, 2004), xxvi, 11.

13. Glenmullen, *Prozac Backlash*, 156–159, 162–165, 177, 225–226.

14. M. Weaver, "Psychiatrists Shift the Mood on Antidepressants," *Society Guardian* (February 2002), accessed at www.society.guardian.co.uk.

15. P. Breggin, M.D., and D. Cohen, Ph.D., *Your Drug May Be Your Problem* (New York: HarperCollins, 1999), 31.

16. Ibid., 106.

17. Glenmullen, *Prozac Backlash*, 211.

18. Ibid., 205–206.

19. Breggin and Cohen, *Your Drug May Be Your Problem*, 16.

20. Glenmullen, *Prozac Backlash*, 94.

21. Ibid., 50.

22. Ibid., 57.

23. Ibid., 20.

24. Breggin and Cohen, *Your Drug May Be Your Problem*, 66.

25. N. Weintrob, et al., "Decreased Growth During Therapy with Selective Serotonin Reuptake Inhibitors," *Archives of Pediatric and Adolescent Medicine* 156, no. 7 (July 2002): 696–701.

26. Ibid., 26.

27. Glenmullen, *Prozac Backlash*, 14.

28. Ibid., 24, 34.

29. A. Montejo-Gonzalez, et al., "SSRI-Induced Sexual Dysfunction," *Journal of Sex and Marital Therapy* 23, no. 3 (Fall 1997): 176–194.

30. *Physician's Drug Handbook* (Springhouse, PA: Springhouse, 1999), 137, 474, 819, 967.

31. Breggin and Cohen, *Your Drug May Be Your Problem*, 76–81.

32. Ibid., 69.

33. Ibid., 70.

34. *Physician's Drug Handbook*, 632.

35. Breggin and Cohen, *Your Drug May Be Your Problem*, 75.

36. *Practice Guidelines for the Treatment of Psychiatric Disorders* (Washington, DC: American Psychiatric Association, 2000), 511.

37. Breggin and Cohen, *Your Drug May Be Your Problem*, 75–76.

38. Glenmullen, *Prozac Backlash*, 52.

39. T. Kishi and J. K. Elmquist, "Body Weight is Regulated by the Brain," *Molecular Psychiatry* 10, no. 2 (February 2005): 132–146.

40. Breggin and Cohen, *Your Drug May Be Your Problem*, 78.

41. Glenmullen, *Prozac Backlash*, 38.

42. Breggin and Cohen, *Your Drug May Be Your Problem*, 79.

43. Ibid., 71–74.

44. Weaver, "Psychiatrists Shift the Mood on Antidepressants."

45. Breggin and Cohen, *Your Drug May Be Your Problem*, 31.

46. R. W. Licht, et al., "A Lithium Clinic for Bipolar Patients: 2-Year Outcome of the First 148 Patients," *Acta Psychiatrica Scandinavia* 104, no. 5 (November 2001): 387–390.

47. T. Mueller, et al., "Recurrence After Recovery from Major Depressive Disorder During 15 Years of Observational Follow-up," *American Journal of Psychiatry* 156, no. 7 (July 1999): 1000–1006.

48. Montejo-Gonzalez, "SSRI-Induced Sexual Dysfunction," 176–94.

49. Glenmullen, *Prozac Backlash*, 38, 52.

50. Breggin and Cohen, *Your Drug May Be Your Problem*, 61.

51. Ibid., 62.

52. U.S. Food and Drug Administration, Public Health Advisory, March 22, 2004, accessed at www.fda.gov/cder/drug/antidepressants/AntidepressantsPHA.htm.

53. Breggin and Cohen, *Your Drug May Be Your Problem*, 66. Also, Weintrob, "Decreased Growth During Therapy with Selective Serotonin Reuptake Inhibitors," 696–701.

54. S. Dalton, et al., "Antidepressant Medications and Risk for Cancer," *Epidemiology* 11, no. 2 (March 2000): 171–176.

55. B. Harlow, et al., "Psychotropic Medication Use and Risk of Epithelial Ovarian Cancer," *Cancer Epidemiology and Biomarkers Prevention* 7, no. 8 (August 1998): 697–702.

56. C. Alfaro, et al., "CYP2D6 Status of Extensive Metabolizers After Multiple-Dose Fluoxetine, Fluvoxamine, Paroxetine, or Sertraline," *Journal of Clinical Psychopharmacology* 19, no. 2 (April 1999): 155–63. Also, R. Soti, et al., "Genetic Polymorphisms of CYP2D6, GSTMl, and GSTTl Genes and Bladder Cancer Risk in North India," *Cancer Genetics and Cytogenetics* 156, no. 1 (January 2005): 68–73. Also, R. Sobti, et al., "CYP1A1 and CYP2D6 Polymorphism and Risk of Lung Cancer in a North Indian Population," *Biomarkers* 8, no. 5 (September–October 2003): 415–28. Also, W. Shi and S. Chen, "Frequencies of Poor Metabolizers of Cytochrome P450 2C19 in Esophagus Cancer, Stomach Can-

cer, Lung Cancer and Bladder Cancer in Chinese Population," *World Journal of Gastroenterology* 10, no. 13 (July 2004): 1961–1963.

57. H. Cohen, et al., "Excess Risk of Myocardial Infarction in Patients Treated with Antidepressant Medications: Association with Use of Tricyclic Agents," *American Journal of Medicine* 108, no. 1 (January 2000): 2–8.

58. J. Silvestre and J. Prous, "Research on Adverse Drug Events. I. Muscarinic M(3) Receptor Binding Affinity Could Predict the Risk of Antipsychotics to Induce Type 2 Diabetes," *Methods and Findings in Experimental & Clinical Pharmacology* 27, no. 5 (June 2005): 289–304.

59. P. Gerber and L. Lynd, "Selective Serotonin-Reuptake-Inhibitor-Induced Movement Disorders," *Annals of Pharmacotherapy* 32, no. 6 (June 1998): 692–98. Also, Breggin and Cohen, *Prozac Backlash*, 34–40.

Chapter 1

1. Carl Pfeiffer, Ph.D., M.D., *Nutrition and Mental Illness* (Rochester, VT: Healing Arts Press, 1987), 36.

2. Pharmax LLC, 1239 120th Avenue NE, Suite B, Bellevue, WA 98005. (425) 467–8054, www.pharmaxllc.com.

3. www.emedicine.com/med/topic229.htm.

4. Testimony of Dr. Elias Zerhouni, director, National Institutes of Health, April 1, 2004, reported at www.hhs.gov/budget/testify.

5. http://ucsdnews.ucsd.edu/newsrel/health/Mol%20Psy%;20GRK3.htm.

6. M. Tsuang, et al., "Assessing the Validity of Blood-Based Gene Expression Profiles for the Classification of Schizophrenia and Bipolar Disorder: a Preliminary Report." *American Journal of Medicine Genet B Neuropsychiatr Genet* 133, no. 1 (February 5, 2005): 1–5.

7. J. Challem, *Feed Your Genes Right* (Hoboken, NJ: John Wiley, 2005), 10.

8. Ibid., xiv.

9. Pfeiffer Treatment Center/Health Research Institute, 4575 Weaver Pkwy., Warrenville, IL 60555, (630) 505–0300, www.hriptc.org

10. W. McGinnis, M.D., "Pyroluria: Hidden Cause of Schizophrenia, Bipolar, Depression, and Anxiety symptoms" (May 21, 2004), reported at www.alternativementalhealth.com/articles/pyroluria.htm.

11. G. Kirschmann and J. Kirschmann, *Nutrition Almanac* (New York: McGraw-Hill, 1996), 56, 139.

12. Pyroluria urine testing is done at Bio Center Lab, Wichita, KS, (800) 494-7785.

13. Dr. C. Kraus, Dr. R. Faurie, and Dr. L. Thomas, "Methylation Maintenance," *Functional Foods & Nutraceuticals* (January 2004): 34–36.

14. Challem, *Feed Your Genes Right*, 12.

15. Ibid., 4–5.

16. D. Kiefer, "SAMe," *Life Extension* (January 2005): 68.

17. J. Braly and P. Holford, *The H-Factor Solution*, accessed at www.trans4mind.com, April 19, 2005.

18. "A Simplified Description of DNA Methylation," accessed at www.dnamethsoc.server101.com, April 19, 2005.

19. J. Shamp, "Scientists Search for Remote Control for Altered Genes," *Durham (North Carolina) Herald Sun* (November 2, 2005).

20. "SAM-e Same as Drugs," *Functional Foods & Nutraceuticals* (December 2002): 6.

21. S. Marohn, *The Natural Medicine Guide to Bipolar Disorder* (Charlottesville, VA: Hampton Roads, 2003), 102–104.

22. TMG made from beets is available from Kirkman Laboratories, Lake Oswego, Oregon, (800) 245-8282, www.kirkmanlabs.com.

23. W. Walsh, Ph.D., "Three Most Common Causes of Bipolar Disorder," accessed at www.alternativementalhealth.com/articles/three.htm, April 19, 2005.

24. S. D. Shorvon, et al., "The Neuropsychiatry of Megaloblastic Anaemia." *British Medical Journal* 281 (1980): 1036–1038.

25. Marohn, *Natural Medicine Guide*, 106–108.

26. A. Cranney, M. Zarkadas, I. Graham, and C. Switzer, "The Canadian Celiac Health Survey," *Biomedical Central Gastroenterology* 3, no. 1 (May 2003): 8.

27. M. Jones, B. Elkus, J. Lyles, and L. Lewis, "Questions and Answers on HLA Typing and Celiac Disease," accessed at www.enabling.org, April 22, 2005.

Chapter 2

1. www.truehope.com, (888) 878–3467.
2. www.quietminds.us.
3. Kirschmann and Kirschmann, *Nutrition Almanac*, 46.
4. J. Balch, M.D., and P. Balch, C.N.C., *Prescription for Nutritional Healing* (New York: Penguin Putnam, 1997), 15.
5. M. Lesser, M.D., *The Brain Chemistry Diet* (New York: Penguin Putnam, 2002), 71–75.
6. Balch and Balch, *Prescription for Nutritional Healing*, 53–54.
7. "A Nutrient Protocol Based on a Research Approach to the Treatment of Mental Disorders," accessed at www.truehope.com, August 6, 2003 revision, "The Use of Empowerplus," 12.
8. Kirschmann and Kirschmann, *Nutrition Almanac*, 59–62.
9. Ibid., 63–64.
10. Ibid., 33–39.
11. *Disease Prevention and Treatment* (Hollywood, FL: Life Extension, 2003), 695.
12. Kirschmann and Kirschmann, *Nutrition Almanac*, 81–84.
13. "Science Update," *Functional Foods & Nutraceuticals* (July/August 2003): 30.
14. Kirschmann and Kirschmann, *Nutrition Almanac*, 103–106.
15. "A Nutrient Protocol Based on a Research Approach to the Treatment of Mental Disorders," accessed at www.truehope.com, August 6, 2003 revision, "The Use of Empowerplus," 26.
16. Kirschmann and Kirschmann, *Nutrition Almanac*, 111.
17. Lesser, *The Brain Chemistry Diet*, 264.
18. A. Bruner, et al., "Randomised Study of Cognitive Effects of Iron Supplementation in Non-Anaemic Iron-Deficient Adolescent Girls," *Lancet* 1996; 348: 973, 992–996.
19. "A Nutrient Protocol Based on a Research Approach to the Treatment of Mental Disorders," accessed at www.truehope.com, August 6, 2003 revisions, "The Use of Empowerplus," 20.
20. C. Dean, M.D., N.D., *The Miracle of Magnesium* (New York: Ballantine, 2003), 51.
21. "A Nutrient Protocol Based on a Research Approach to the Treatment of Mental Disorders," 29.

22. Kirschmann and Kirschmann, *Nutrition Almanac*, 129–131.

23. *Life Extension* (December 2004): 48.

24. Kirschmann and Kirschmann, *Nutrition Almanac*, 139–141.

25. P. Renshaw, "Cheering Chow," *Harvard Magazine*, 17.

26. A. Stoll, M.D., *The Omega-3 Connection* (New York: Simon & Schuster, 2001).

27. C. Hosmer, M.S., R.D., "Ask the Doctor," *Harvard Heart Letter* (November 2005): 8.

28. U. Erasmus Ph.D., *Fats that Heal, Fats that Kill* (Burnaby, BC, Canada: Alive Books, 1993), 125–127.

Chapter 3

1. "How Biomagnetism Works," reported at www.naturalfeeling.com, accessed March 23, 2005.

2. S. Leighton, M.D., Family Care Health & Wellness Center, (336) 723-9002.

3. D. Papolos, M.D., and J. Papolos, *The Bipolar Child* (New York: Broadway Books, 1999), 34–35.

4. G. Cousens, M.D., *Depression-Free for Life* (New York: HarperCollins, 2000), 29.

5. "The Physical Causes of Depression," accessed at www.alternativemental health.com/articles, March 23, 2005.

6. J. Strohecker, et al., *Natural Healing for Depression* (New York: Penguin Putnam, 1999), 55.

7. Ibid., 134–135.

8. *Alternative Medicine: The Definitive Guide* (Fife, WA: Future Medicine, 1995), 936.

9. L. Chaitow, et al., *Fibromyalgia Syndrome: A Practitioner's Guide to Treatment* (London: Harcourt Publishers, 2000), 69.

10. D. Cole, et al., "Slower Treatment Response in Bipolar Depression Predicted by Lower Pretreatment Thyroid Function," *American Journal of Psychiatry* 159, no. 1 (January 2002): 116–21.

11. *Life Extension Disease Prevention and Treatment* (Hollywood, FL: Life Extension, 2003), 1551.

12. E. Wilson, M.D., *Wilson's Thyroid Syndrome* (Lady Lake, FL: WilsonsThyroidSyndrome.com, 2001), 111.

13. *Life Extension Disease Prevention and Treatment*, 1545.

14. I. Ekimova, "Changes in the Metabolic Activity of Neurons in the Anterior Hypothalamic Nuclei in Rats During Hyperthermia, Fever, and Hypothermia," *Neuroscience and Behavioral Physiology* 33, no. 5 (June 2003): 455–460.

15. www.wilsonsthyroidsyndrome.com, accessed July 14, 2004.

16. S. Refetoff, et al., "The Syndromes of Resistance to Thyroid Hormone" *Endocrine Review* 14 (1993): 348–399.

17. Specially compounded T_3 is available from Mountain View Pharmacy, 10565 N. Tatum Blvd., #B-118, Paradise Valley, AZ 85253, (800) 942–7065 or (480) 948–7065; fax 480–948–9489, Evelyn D. Timmons, FACA, FIACP, pharmacist.

18. M. Milner, "Wilson's Syndrome and T_3 Therapy," *International Journal of Pharmaceutical Compounding* 3, no. 5 (1999): 344–348.

19. *Life Extension Disease Prevention and Treatment*, 1550.

20. J. Lee, M.D., *What Your Doctor May Not Tell You About Breast Cancer* (New York: Warner Books, 2002), 218.

21. *Life Extension* magazine, Collector's Edition (2005): 25.

22. N. Tagawa, et al., "Seru Dehydroepiandrosterone, Dehydroepiandosterone Sulfate, and Pregnenolone Sulfate Concentrations in Patients with Hyperthyroidism and Hypothyroidism," *Clinical Chemistry* 46, no. 4 (April 2000): 523–528.

23. E. Barret-Connor, et al., "A Prospective Study of Dehydroepiandrosterone Sulfate, Mortality and Cardiovascular Disease," *New England Journal of Medicine* 315 (December 11, 1986): 1519–1524.

24. K. Dhatarigy, et al., "Effect of Dehydroepiandrosterone Replacement on Insulin Sensitivity and Lipids in Hypoadrenal Women," *Diabetes* 54, no. 3 (March 2005): 765–769. Also, D. Villareal and J. Holloszy, "Effect of DHEA on Abdominal Fat and Insulin Action in Elderly Women and Men: A Randomized Controlled Trial," *Journal of the American Medical Association* 292, no. 18 (November 10, 2004): 2243–2248.

25. D. Young, N.D., *Essential Oils* (Lehi, UT: Essential Science Publications, 2003), 388; www.essentialscience.net.

26. J. Ross, M.A., *The Mood Cure* (New York: Penguin Group, 2002), 94.

27. D. Khalsa, M.D., *Brain Longevity* (New York: Warner Books, 1997), 39–40.
28. S. Strogatz, *Sync* (New York: Hyperion, 2003), 82–89.
29. U. Reiss, M.D./OB-Gyn, *Natural Hormone Balance for Women* (New York: Simon & Schuster, 2001), 206–207.
30. Ross, *The Mood Cure*, 238–239.
31. J. Brody, "Scientists Find Ways to Reset Biological Clocks in Dim Winter," *The New York Times* Health (December 29, 1993).
32. J. Lee, M.D., *What Your Doctor May Not Tell You About Menopause* (New York: Warner Books, 1996), 50–58.
33. Reiss, *Natural Hormone Balance for Women*, 93.
34. Lesser, *The Brain Chemistry Diet*, 264.
35. Lee, *What Your Doctor May Not Tell You About Menopause*, 50–58.
36. Ibid., 146–147.
37. Ibid., 12, 126.
38. Reiss, *Natural Hormone Balance for Women*, 6–7.
39. K. Weier and M. Beal, "Complementary Therapies as Adjuncts in the Treatment of Postpartum Depression." *Journal of Midwifery and Women's Health* 49, no. 2 (March–April 2004): 96–104.
40. Reiss, *Natural Hormone Balance for Women*, 158–159.
41. Ibid., 168, 171.

Chapter 4

1. N. Moore, Ph.D., Life Coaching Institute, 4009 Old Denton Rd., Carrollton, TX 75007, (214) 739–6644, www.drneecie.com.
2. Mannatech, 600 S. Royal Lane, #200, Coppell, TX 75019, (800) 281–4469, www.mannatech.com.
3. A. Somersall, Ph.D., M.N.D., editor, *The Healing Power of 8 Sugars* (Mississauga, Ontario, Canada: Natural Wellness, 2005), 7, 10–11.
4. S. Nugent, N.D., "The Nugent Toxin Report," reported at www.studentsforlife.net, 9, June 2, 2005.
5. I. MacRobert, M.D., "Taking Back Control of Your Health," reported at www.studentsforlife.net, June 2, 2005.
6. R. Elkins, M.H., *Miracle Sugars* (Orem, UT: Woodland, 2003), 11.

7. Somersall, *The Healing Power of 8 Sugars*, 40.

8. Ibid., 64.

9. Ibid., 286.

10. E. Mondoa, M.D., and M. Kitei, *Sugars That Heal* (New York: Random House, 2001), 113.

11. Somersall, *The Healing Power of 8 Sugars*, 287.

12. Elkins, *Miracle Sugars*, 19.

13. Mondoa and Kitei, *Sugars That Heal*, 24.

14. Somersall, *The Healing Power of 8 Sugars*, 287.

15. Ibid., 288.

16. Ibid.

17. Mondoa and Kitei, *Sugars That Heal*, 24.

18. Ibid., 25.

19. Somersall, *The Healing Power of 8 Sugars*, 289.

20. Elkins, *Miracle Sugars*, 30.

21. Mondoa and Kitei, *Sugars That Heal*, 26.

22. Elkins, *Miracle Sugars*, 37–40.

23. Ibid., 186.

24. M. Zesiewicz, et al., "Effects of Glyconutritional Supplements in Children with Bipolar Disorder," *Proceedings* 4, no. 1 (March 2005): 10–11.

25. Balch and Balch, *Prescription for Nutritional Healing*, 39–42.

26. J. Whitaker, M.D., *Dr. Whitaker's Guide to Natural Healing* (Rocklin, CA: Prima, 1996), 317.

27. Lee, *What Your Doctor May Not Tell You About Menopause*, 178–179.

28. Balach and P. Balach, *Prescription for Nutritional Healing*, 42.

29. M. Murray, N.D., and J. Pizzorno, N.D., *Encyclopedia of Natural Medicine* (Rocklin, CA: Prima, 1998), 391.

30. Ibid., 394–395.

31. *Amino Acid Connection* (San Francisco: Pax Publications, 1985), an amino acid poster.

32. Balch and Balch, *Prescription for Nutritional Healing*, 37.

33. Ibid., 41.

34. Murray and Pizzorno, *Encyclopedia of Natural Medicine*, 393.

35. Balch and Balch, *Prescription for Nutritional Healing*, 41.

36. Ibid., 42.

37. A. Pressman, D.C., Ph.D., C.C.N., *Glutathione: The Ultimate Antioxidant* (New York: St. Martin's Press, 1997), 168.
38. Balch and Balch, *Prescription for Nutritional Healing*, 38.
39. E. Edelman, *Natural Healing for Schizophrenia* (Eugene, OR: Borage Books, 2001), 145.
40. Pressman, *Glutathione*, 4–6.
41. www.moodcure.com/aminoacidprecautions.html, accessed September 2005.
42. Kirschmann and Kirschmann, *Nutrition Almanac*, 389–469.

Chapter 5

1. Sukyo Mahikari Center, 72 Madison Ave., 4th Floor, New York, NY, (212) 447–5811.
2. Marohn, *The Natural Medicine Guide*, 142.
3. www.naet.com.
4. L. Davidson, C. Harding, and L. Spaniol, eds., *Recovery from Severe Mental Illnesses* (Boston: Center for Psychiatric Rehabilitation, Boston University, 2005), 6.
5. S. Walker III, M.D., *A Dose of Sanity* (Hoboken, NJ: John Wiley, 1997).
6. E. Klonoff and H. Landrine, *Preventing Misdiagnosis of Women: A Guide to Physical Disorders That Have Psychiatric Symptoms* (London: Sage, 1997).
7. S. Weintraub, N.D., *Allergies and Holistic Healing* (Pleasant Grove, UT: Woodland Publishing, 1997), 17.
8. E. Lipski, M.S., C.C.N., *Digestive Wellness* (Lincolnwood, IL: Keats, 2000), 104.
9. M. Gershon, M.D., *The Second Brain* (New York: HarperCollins, 1998), xii–xiii.
10. R. Lydiard, et al., "Prevalence of Psychiatric Disorders in Patients with Irritable Bowel Syndrome," *Psychosomatics* 34, no. 3 (May–June 1993): 229–234.
11. Kirschmann and Kirschmann, *Nutrition Almanac*, 307.
12. K. DeFelice, *Enzymes for Autism and Other Neurological Conditions* (Johnston, IA: kjorn@thundersnow.com, 2003), 114.
13. Loomis Institute of Enzyme Nutrition, 6421 Enterprise Lane, Madison, WI 53719, (800) 662–2630, www.loomisenzymes.com.

14. L. Lee, Ph.D., "The Effects of Enzymes on Mental Health," reported at www.alternativementalhealth.com/articles, accessed July 14, 2004.

15. Ibid.

16. L. Lee, Ph.D., 4826 Mahalo Dr., Eugene, OR 97405, (541) 431–1099, www.litalee.com.

17. DeFelice, *Enzymes for Autism*, 78.

18. Houston Nutraceuticals, Inc., P.O. Box 6331, Siloam Springs, AR 72761, (866) 757–8627, www.houstonni.com.

19. D. Charney, et al., "Increased Anxiogenic Effects of Caffeine in Panic Disorders," *Archives of General Psychiatry* 42 (1984): 233–243.

20. S. Bolton and G. Null, "Caffeine, Psychological Effects, Use, and Abuse," *Journal of Orthomolecular Psychiatry* 10 (1981): 202–211.

21. K. Kreitsch, et al., "Prevalence, Presenting Symptoms, and Psychological Characteristics of Individuals Experiencing a Diet-Related Mood Disturbance," *Behavioral Therapy* 19 (1985): 593–594.

22. L. Christensen, "Psychological Distress and Diet: Effects of Sucrose and Caffeine," *Journal of Applied Nutrition* 40 (1988): 44–50.

23. D'Adamo, *Eat Right 4 Your Type*, 23–24, 67, 111.

24. Great Smokies Diagnostic Laboratory, 63 Zillicoa St., Asheville, NC 28801-1074, www.gsdl.com.

25. Elkins, *Miracle Sugars*, 20–23.

Chapter 6

1. "Report 13 of the Council on Scientific Affairs (A-04)," February 25, 2005, accessed at www.ama-assn.org.

2. J. Gorman, "Does Mercury Matter?" *New York Times* (July 29, 2003): D5.

3. C. Leong, et al., "Retrograde Degeneration of Neurite Membrane Structural Integrity of Nerve Growth Cones Following *In Vitro* Exposure to Mercury," *NeuroReport* 12, no. 4 (March 26, 2001): 733–737.

4. W. Wolcott and T. Fahey, *The Metabolic Typing Diet* (New York: Doubleday, 2000), 342–346.

5. S. Baker, M.D., *Detoxification and Healing* (New York: McGraw-Hill, 2004), 116.

6. J. Whitaker, M.D., *Dr. Whitaker's Guide to Natural Healing* (Rocklin, CA: Prima, 1996), 76.

7. Ibid., 115.

8. "Copper Toxicity," brochure, Eck Institute of Applied Nutrition and Bioenergetics, Ltd., 2225 W. Alice Ave., Phoenix, AZ 85021, (602) 995–1580.

9. Lesser, *The Brain Chemistry Diet*, 264.

10. The Eck Institute, Depression Newsletter, 17, no. 1 (November 2001).

11. Edelman, *Natural Healing for Schizophrenia*, 38.

12. *Disease Prevention and Treatment* (Hollywood, FL: Life Extension, 2003), 935.

13. Environmental Working Group's Web site, www.ewg.org/reports/bodyburden/es.php, accessed July 15, 2005.

14. C. Stapleton, "Toxic Elements Found in Infants' Cord Blood," *Palm Beach Post* (July 14, 2005).

15. E. Knobil, et al., *Hormonally Active Agents in the Environment* (Washington, DC: National Academy Press, 1999).

16. To order an informative booklet. *Earth Friendly Alternatives to Herbicides, Pesticides, and Household Chemicals*, mail $6 plus $1 postage to: Stonington Garden Club, P.O. Box 385, Stonington, CT 06378; for more info go to www.stonington-gardenclub.org.

17. Murray and Pizzorno, *Encyclopedia of Natural Medicine*, 110–111.

18. Ibid., 113–116.

19. S. Baker, M.D., *Detoxification and Healing* (New York: McGraw-Hill, 2004), 152–159.

20. Great Smokies Diagnostic Laboratory, 63 Zillicoa St., Asheville, NC 28801, www.gsdl.com.

21. S. Rogers, M.D., *Detoxify or Die* (Sarasota, FL: Sand Key, 2002), 149.

22. S. Baker, M.D., *Detoxification and Healing*, 112.

23. High Tech Health, Inc., 2695 Linden Drive, Boulder, CO 80304, www.hightechhealth.com.

24. D. Yance, *Herbal Medicine, Healing & Cancer* (Lincolnwood, IL: Keats, 1999), 202.

Chapter 7

1. Analytical Research Labs, Inc., 2225 W. Alice Ave., Phoenix, AZ 85021, (602) 995–1581, www.arltma.com.
2. Ibid., Analytical Research Labs report to Elena, dated March 8, 2004.
3. Lipski, *Digestive Wellness*, 59–65.
4. Ibid., 61.
5. S. Weintraub, N.D., *Allergies and Holistic Healing* (Pleasant Grove, UT: Woodland, 1997), 139.
6. L. Chaitow, N.D., D.O., *Fibromyalgia Syndrome* (Edinburgh, England: Harcourt, 2000), 180.
7. Whitaker, *Dr. Whitaker's Guide to Natural Healing*, 176–184.
8. W. Crook, M.D., "Hyperactivity and the Yeast Connection," reported at www.latitudes.org, accessed March 9, 2004.
9. Weintraub, *Allergies and Holistic Healing*, 145–146.
10. Ross, *The Mood Cure*, 250–251.
11. J. Strohecker, editor, *Natural Healing for Depression* (New York: Penguin Putnam, 1999), 100.
12. Recovery Systems, 147 Lomita Drive, Suite D, Mill Valley, CA 94941, (415) 383–3611, ext. #1, www.moodcure.com.
13. K. Gilliland and W. Bullick, "Caffeine: A Potential Drug of Abuse," *Advances in Alcohol and Substance Abuse* 3 (1984): 53–73.
14. Bolton and Null, "Caffeine, Psychological Effects Use, and Abuse," 202–211.
15. Murray and Pizzorno, *Encyclopedia of Natural Medicine*, 384.
16. R. Wurtman and J. Wurtman, "Brain Serotonin, Carbohydrate-Craving, Obesity and Depression," *Obesity Research* 3, Supplement 4 (November 1995): 477S–480S.
17. Ross, *The Mood Cure*, 345.
18. "Quarterly Report on Adverse Reactions Associated with Aspartame Ingestion" (Washington, DC: Center for Food Safety and Nutrition, U.S. FDA, April 1, 1988).
19. Ross, *The Mood Cure*, 29.
20. B. Martini, "The Connection between Aspartame and Panic Attacks, Depression, Bipolar Disorder, Memory Problems, and Other Mental

Symptoms," reported at www.alternativementalhealth.com, accessed June 8, 2005.

21. Weintraub, *Allergies and Holistic Healing*, 217–221.
22. Strohecker, *Natural Healing for Depression*, 62.
23. C. Danielson, et al., "Hip Fractures and Fluoridation in Utah's Elderly Population," *Journal of the American Medical Association* 268, no. 6 (August 1992): 746–748.
24. N. Revis, et al., "Relationship of Drinking Water Disinfectants to Plasma Cholesterol and Thyroid Hormone Levels in Experimental Studies," *Proceedings of the National Academy of Sciences of the USA* 8 (1986): 1485–1489.
25. N. Revis, et al., "Relationship of Dietary Iodide and Drinking Water Disinfectants to Thyroid Function in Experimental Animals," *Environmental Health Perspectives* 69 (1986): 243–246.
26. E. Zeighami, et al., "Chlorination, Water Hardness and Serum Cholesterol in Forty-six Wisconsin Communities," *International Journal of Epidemiology* 19 (1990): 49–58.

Chapter 8

1. *Alternative Medicine*, 782.
2. Ibid., 782–784.
3. F. Strick, "The Role of Infections in Mental Illness," reported at www.alternativementalhealth.com, accessed September 22, 2005.
4. A. Brown, et al., "Maternal Exposure to Toxoplasmosis and Risk of Schizophrenia in Adult Offspring," *American Journal of Psychiatry* 162, no. 4 (2005): 767–773.
5. L. Jones-Brando, et al., "Drugs Used in the Treatment of Schizophrenia and Bipolar Disorder Inhibit the Replication of *Toxoplasma gondii*," *Schizophrenia Research* 62, no. 3 (August 1, 2003): 237–244.
6. Strick, "The Role of Infections in Mental Illness."
7. D. Cruess, et al., "Prevalence, Diagnosis, and Pharmacological Treatment of Mood Disorder in HIV Disease," *Biological Psychiatry* 54, no. 3 (August 1, 2003): 307–316.

8. D. Hart, et al., "Antiretroviral Antibodies: Implications for Schizophrenia, Schizophrenia Spectrum Disorders, and Bipolar Disorder," *Biological Psychiatry* 45, no. 6 (March 15, 1999): 704–714.

9. O. Frank, et al., "Human Endogenous Retrovirus Expression Profiles in Samples from Brains of Patients with Schizophrenia and Bipolar Disorders," *Journal of Virology* 79, no. 17 (September 2005): 10890–108901.

10. J. Talan, "Animal Virus May Play a Role in Some Mental Disorders," *Newsday* Feature Reported in the *Providence Sunday Journal* (November 30, 1997).

11. H. Terayama, et al., "Detection of Anti-Borna Disease Virus Antibodies from Patients with Schizophrenia and Mood Disorders in Japan," *Psychiatry Research* 120, no. 2 (September 30, 2003): 201–206.

12. D'Adamo, *Eat Right 4 Your Type*, 98, 288.

Chapter 9

1. V. Ibric, M.D., Ph.D., B.C.I.A.C., D.A.B.P.S., Therapy and Prevention Center, 65 N. Madison Ave., #450, Pasadena, CA 91101, (626) 577–2202, www.neurofeedback-dribric.com.

2. Ross, *The Mood Cure* and *The Diet Cure* (New York: Penguin Books, 2002).

3. Recovery Systems, 147 Lomita Drive, Suite D, Mill Valley, CA 94941, (415) 383–3611, www.moodcure.com.

4. H. Mann, M.D., psychiatrist and neurofeedback practitioner, 188 Wolf Neck Road, Stonington, CT 06378, (860) 536–6023, personal communication, October 2005.

5. S. Garland, "Biofeedback Moves Toward the Mainstream," *Business Week* (October 16, 2000).

6. Mann, personal communication, October 2005.

7. B. McAnnalley, et al., "An Interpretation of the Effects of a Single Dose of a Glyconutritional Supplement on the Brain Function of Healthy College Students, Including a Review of Brainwave Function," *Glyco-Science and Nutrition* 3, no. 4 (July 1, 2002).

8. Mann, personal communication, October 2005.

9. Ibid.

10. Ibid.

11. Ibid.

12. McAnnalley, "An Interpretation of the Effects of a Single Dose of a Glyconutritional Supplement."

13. EEG Institute is the clinic and research center of the Brian Othmer Foundation, 22020 Clarendon Street, #305, Woodland Hills, CA 91361, www.eegsupport.com.

14. A. Oubry, Ph.D., "EEG Neurofeedback for Treating Psychiatric Disorders," *Psychiatric Times* XIX, no. 2 (February 2002).

15. A.D.D. Institute, "Neurofeedback and Depression," reported at www.hp-add.com/depress.htm, accessed July 21, 2004.

16. LENs system Web site: www.ochlabs.com/intro.php with link to providers.

17. Mann, personal communication, October 2005.

18. D. Hammond, Ph.D., "Neurofeedback for Depression," reported at www.isnr.org/pubarea/depression.htm, accessed September 27, 2005.

Chapter 10

1. Equilib is manufactured by Evince International, (866) 437–7093, www.equilib.us.

2. www.emdr.com.

3. "A List of Major Psychological Sequelae of Abortion," reported at www.afterabortion.info/psychol.html, accessed November 1, 2005.

4. *American College of Physicians Complete Home Medical Guide* (New York: DK Publishing, 1999), 510.

5. D. Servan-Schreiber, M.D., Ph.D., *The Instinct to Heal* (Emmaus, PA: Rodale Press, 2004), 25.

6. D. Khalsa, M.D., *Brain Longevity* (New York: Warner Books, 1997), 110–112.

7. G. Ironson, et al., "Comparison of Two Treatments for Traumatic Stress: A Community-Based Study of EMDR and Exposure," *Journal of Clinical Psychiatry* 58 (2002): 113–128.

8. M. Van Etten and S. Taylor, "Comparative Efficacy of Treatments for Posttraumatic Stress Disorder: A Meta-Analysis," *Clinical Psychology and Psychotherapy* 5 (1998): 126–144.

9. S. Sartori and R. Poirrier, "Seasonal Affective Syndrome and Phototherapy: Theoretical Concepts and Clinical Applications," *Encaphale* 22, no. 1 (January–February 1996): 7–16.

10. Ibid.,

11. M. Rao, et al., "Blood Serotonin, Serum Melatonin and Light Therapy in Healthy Subjects and in Patients with Nonseasonal Depression," *Acta Psychiatrica Scandinavia* 86, no. 2 (August 1992): 127–132.

12. K. Rohan, et al, "Cognitive-Behavioral Therapy, Light Therapy, and Their Combination in Treating Seasonal Affective Disorder," *Journal of Affective Disorders* 80, nos. 2–3 (June 2004): 273–283.

13. M. Hutchison, *Mega Brain* (New York: Ballantine Books, 1991).

14. Rohan, "Cognitive-Behavioral Therapy, Light Therapy, and Their Combination in Treating Seasonal Affective Disorder," 273–283.

15. S. Vazquez, Ph.D., "The New Light Psychotherapy for Seasonal Affective Disorder (SAD)," *Journal of American Psychotherapy* (Fall 2004): 18–26.

16. S. Vazquez, Ph.D., "A New Paradigm for PTSD Treatment: Emotional Transformation Therapy," *Journal of American Psychotherapy* (Summer 2004): 20–26.

Chapter 11

1. L. Hay, *You Can Heal Your Life* (Carlsbad, CA: Hay House, 1984), www.hayhouse.com.

2. G. Epstein, M.D., American Institute for Mental Imagery, 16 East 96th St., #1A, New York, NY 10128, (212) 369–4080, www.drjerryepstein.org.

3. D. Khalsa, M.D., *Brain Longevity* (New York: Warner Books, 1997), 324–325.

4. G. Brainard, et al., "Plasma Cortisol Reduction in Healthy Volunteers Following a Single Yoga Session of Yoga Practices," *Yoga Research Society Newsletter* (Philadelphia: Neurology Department, Jefferson Medical College, 1997), no. 18.

5. E. Hoffman, Ph.D., "Mapping the Brain's Activity after Kriya Yoga," www.scan-Yoga.org.

6. A. Weintraub, *Yoga for Depression* (New York: Broadway Books, 2004), 151–154.

7. R. Brown and P. Gerberg, "Sudarshan Kriya Yogic Breathing in the Treatment of Stress, Anxiety, and Depression: Part II—Clinical Applications and Guidelines," *Journal of Alternative and Complementary Medicine* 11, no. 4 (August 2005): 711–717.

8. Weintraub, *Yoga for Depression*, 156.

9. Ibid., 171–178.

10. O. Mason and I. Hargreaves, "A Qualitative Study of Mindfulness-Based Cognitive Therapy for Depression," *British Journal of Medical Psychology* 74, Part 2 (June 2001): 197–212.

11. D. Shannahoff-Khalsa, "An Introduction to Kundalini Yoga Meditation Techniques that are Specific for the Treatment of Psychiatric Disorders," *Journal of Alternative and Complementary Medicine* 10, no. 1 (February 2004): 91–101.

12. P. Barnes, et al., "Complementary and Alternative Medicine Use Among Adults: United States, 2002," *Advanced Data* 343 (May 27, 2004): 1–19.

13. "Guide to Relieving Stress," Harvard Health Publications (President & Fellows of Harvard College, 2002), 3.

14. R. D'Souza and A. Rodrigo, "Spiritually Augmented Cognitive Behavioural Therapy," *Australas Psychiatry* 12, no. 2 (June 2004): 148–152.

15. H. Benson, M.D., *Timeless Healing* (New York: Fireside, 1997), 20–22.

16. C. Myss, Ph.D., *Anatomy of the Spirit* (New York: Crown, 1996), 47–48.

Chapter 12

1. J. Adams, Adams Healing Arts, 15 Church St., Mystic, CT 06355, (860) 572-9341, www.adamshealingarts.com.

2. R. Gerber, M.D., *Vibrational Medicine* (Rochester, VT: Bear & Co., 2001), 24.

3. C. Weze, et al., "Evaluation of Healing by Gentle Touch," *Public Health* 119, no. 1 (January 2005): 3–10.

4. D. Eden, *Energy Medicine* (New York: Penguin Putnam, 1998), 172–173.

5. Gerber, *Vibrational Medicine*, 51–52.

6. Ibid., 53.

7. B. Brennan, *Hands of Light* (New York: Bantam Books, 1987).

8. Barbara Brennan School of Healing, 500 NE Spanish River Blvd., #208, Boca Raton, Florida 33431, www.barbarabrennan.com.

9. Harvard Heart Letter (October 2005).

10. Gerber, *Vibrational Medicine*, 122–123.

11. *Alternative Medicine*, 38.

12. Ibid., 40–41.

13. H. MacPherson, et al., "Acupuncture for Depression: First Steps Toward a Clinical Evaluation," *Journal of Alternative and Complementary Medicine* 10, no. 6 (December 2004): 1083–1091.

14. A. Shore, "Long-Term Effects of Energetic Healing on Symptoms of Psychological Depression and Self-Perceived Stress," *Alternative Therapies in Health and Medicine* 10, no. 4 (July–August 2004): 14.

15. D. Vennells, *Reiki for Beginners* (St. Paul, MN: Llewellyn Worldwide, 1999), 9–35.

16. B. Rogers, Stonebridge Herbary, Olde Mystic Village, #15, Mystic, CT 06355, (860) 572–9545.

17. E. Brown, Center for Pain Relief, 94 N. Anguilla Rd., Pawcatuck, CT 06379, (860) 599–3373.

18. D. Chopra, M.D., *The Spontaneous Fulfillment of Desire* (New York: Random House, 2003).

Chapter 13

1. Dee Cee Laboratories, White House, TN 37188, www.Formula303.com. Order via The Wellness Emporium, (702) 362–2776.

2. Oasis Life Sciences, 2660 Willamette Drive NE, Lacey, WA 98516, (360) 486–7500, www.npros.com.

3. www.bodytalksystem.com.

4. K. Hope, Radiant Action, 3234 NE Wasco, St., Portland, OR 97232, (503) 230–2700.

5. www.renresearch.com.

6. A. Lansky, Ph.D., *Impossible Cure* (Portola Valley, CA: R. L. Ranch Press, 2003), 24–29, www.impossiblecure.com.

7. Ibid., 29–30.

8. Ibid., 4.

9. T. Fior, M.D., A.B.F.P., D.Ht., "A Fact Sheet on Homeopathy," reported at www.citizens.org/news/newsletter/2005/november/articles.

10. Lansky, *Impossible Cure*, 180–181.

11. D. Ullman, "Controlled Clinical Trials Evaluating the Homeopathic Treatment of People with Human Immunodeficiency Virus or Acquired Immune Deficiency Syndrome," *Journal of Alternative and Complementary Medicine* 9, no. 1 (February 2003): 133–141.

12. I. Bell, et al., "Improved Clinical Status in Fibromyalgia Patients Treated with Individualized Homeopathic Remedies Versus Placebo," *Rheumatology* (Oxford) 43, no. 5 (May 2004): 577–582; Epub January 20, 2004.

Chapter 14

1. A. Stoll, M.D., *The Omega-3 Connection* (New York: Simon & Schuster, 2001), 214.

2. Glenmullen, *Prozac Backlash*, 74.

Index

acetylcholine, 10
acidophilus, 125
acupuncture, 188, 190, 191–92
Adams, Jill, 184–85, 187–88
ADHD, 7–8
adrenal hormones, 70
affirmations, 171–72, 177–79
alcohol, 129
allergens, 97–98
allergies, 90–105
    case study, 90–97
    categories of reactions, 98
    causes of, 97–98
    diagnosis and elimination,
        103–5
    digestion and, 98–102
    food allergy triggers, 103
Allergies and Holistic Healing
    (Weintraub), 132
allopathic medicine, 201–2
alpha-linolenic acid (ALA), 58
alpha waves, 155, 180
alternative therapies, increasing use
    of, 21–24
aluminum, 115
Alzheimer's disease, 8–9

American Journal of Psychiatry, 142
American Medical Association, 201,
    202
*American Psychiatric Association
    Practice Guidelines*, 18, 164
amino acids, 81
    eight essential, 85–89
    supplementation, 89, 217–18
amygdala, 165
amylase, 100
Anatomy of the Spirit (Myss), 183
Angell, Marcia, 13
Annals of Internal Medicine, 68
antibodies (immunoglobulins),
    97–98
antidepressants. *see* psychiatric drugs
antigens, 97
anti-inflammatory diet, 223–25
arachidonic acid, 28, 223
arsenic, 114
ascorbic acid (vitamin C), 53
aspartame, 131–32
attention deficit hyperactivity
    disorder (ADHD), 7–8
auras, 188, 189
author's story, 2–4, 27–33

bacteria, beneficial, 125–26
Baker, Sidney, 119–20
Beecher, Henry K., 183
Benson, Herbert, 182
Bernard, Claude, 12
beta-carotene, 53
beta waves, 154
bifidus (*bifidobacterium*), 126
bingeing and purging, 136–37,
    138–39, 140
biofeedback, 153–54
biotin, 52–53, 228
bipolar disorder
    author's story, 2–4, 27–33
    occurrence of, 1–2
    symptoms and diagnosis, 4, 6–7
    vs. ADHD in children, 7–8
birth control pills, 73–74
Bishop, Kassidi (case study), 44–50
Blastocystic hominis, 140–41
body burden, 117
BodyTalk, 198–99
body temperature, 68–69, 72
borna virus, 143
boron, 54
Boudreau, Tracy (case study), 207–14
brain
    minerals and, 54–57
    mood disorders and, 9–11
    neurofeedback, 149–57
    parts of, 165
    substances that disrupt, 129–35
    technology for observation of, 4
    violence and, 36
    vitamins and, 50–54
Brain Longevity (Khalsa), 71, 181

brain waves, 153–57, 180
Breiner, Mark A., 112
Brennan, Barbara A., 189, 194
British Medical Journal, 203
Brown, Ellie, 194
bulimia, 136–37, 138–39, 140
Burk, Dean, 135
Burr, Harold S., 189
B-vitamins, 50–53

cadmium, 114–15
caffeine, 103, 129–30
calcium, 54–55, 105
Candida albicans (yeast), 122–29,
    142
    case study, 122–25
    die-off reactions, 128–29
    diets and supplements, 127–29,
        227–32
    symptoms, 126–29
carbohydrases, 100
carbohydrates, 225
carotenes, 53
case studies
    author's story, 2–4, 27–33
    Bishop, Kassidi, 44–50
    Boudreau, Tracy, 207–14
    Elena, 122–25
    Gina, 158–63
    Green, Steven, 106–12
    Hartford, Haley, 77–80
    Jensen, Mary, 90–97
    Joy, 60–65
    Nicole, 149–52
    Raineau, Lindsae, 184–87
    Schmook, Andrea, 170–77

Suzy, 196–99
   Vickie, 136–41
celiac disease, 42–43
cellular thyroid resistance, 68–69
cellulase, 100
cerebrum, 165
Chaitow, Leon, 127
chakras, 189–91
Challem, Jack, 35
chelation, 110, 111
chi, 188, 191
chicken pox virus, 47
children
   ADD drugs and, 16
   ADHD *vs.* bipolar disorder,
      7–8
   antidepressants and, 16
   candida overgrowth, 127
Chirozyme formulas, 101
chocolate, 102–3, 134–35
cholesterol, 74–75
Chopra, Deepak, 194
chromium, 55
cobalamin (vitamin B$_{12}$), 52
coenzyme Q$_{10}$, 105
coenzymes (B-vitamins), 50–53
Combat Fung, 227–28
Commonweal, 117
copper, 41–42, 55, 106, 115–16
cortex, 165
cortisol, 71–72
Crook, William G., 127
Cryptosporidium, 142
CT (computerized tomography),
   4
Cullen, William, 201

cysteine, 87, 218
cystine, 87, 218

D'Adamo, Peter J., 144
Dean, H. Trendley, 135
DeFelice, Karen, 102
delta waves, 155
depression
   causes of, 65–66, 66
   occurrence of, 1
   symptoms and diagnosis, 4–9
detoxification, 109–11, 118–21
Detoxification and Healing (Baker),
   119–20
DHA, 58
DHEA, 70–71
Dientamoeba fragilus, 141–42
digestion, 98–102
   beneficial bacteria, 125–26
   enzyme supplementation, 101–2
   food cravings, 102–3, 130–31
   immune system and, 99–100
   mental illness and, 98–99
   primary enzymes, 100
   process of, 99
   raw *vs.* processed foods, 100–101
Digestive Wellness (Lipski), 125
diphenhydramine, 60
disaccharidases, 100
DMPS, 110
DMSA, 120
DNA, 15, 38
docosahexaenoic acid (DHA), 58
doctors, finding, 214–16
dopamine, 10
downregulation, 15

Dr. Whitaker's Guide to Natural Healing (Whitaker), 127
drugs. *see also* psychiatric drugs
  depression-causing, 66
  mania-causing, 67
dysthymia, 5

EFAs, 57–59
Ehrlich, Paul, 12
eicosapentaenoic acid (EPA), 32, 58–59
electrical fields, 189
Elena (case study), 122–25
EMDR, 162–67
Emotional Transformation Therapy (ETT), 167–69
EMPowerplus, 47–48, 49
energy medicines/therapies, 184–95
  acupuncture, 188, 190, 191–92
  case study, 184–87
  chakras, 189–91
  flow of energy, 188–91
  reiki, 188, 190, 192–93
  therapeutic touch, 187–88, 190, 193–95
  types of, 194
Entamoeba histolytica, 141
Environmental Working Group, 117
The Enzyme Cure (Lee), 101
enzymes, 81, 99–102
Enzymes for Autism (DeFelice), 102
EPA, 32, 58–59
Epstein, Gerald, 179, 180
Equilib, 163, 164
essential fatty acids (EFAs), 57–59

estrogen, 73–74
ETT, 167–69
exercise, 180–81
eye movement desensitization & reprocessing (EMDR), 162–67

far infrared saunas, 120
fatty acids. *see* essential fatty acids (EFAs)
Feed Your Genes Right (Challem), 35
fibromyalgia, 62–65, 127
Fibromyalgia Syndrome (Chaitow), 127
fish consumption and mercury, 113
fish oil supplements, 32–33, 58–59, 216–17
5-HTP, 86–87, 131
fluoride, 135
folic acid (folate, vitamin B_9), 41, 52
Food and Drug Administration (FDA), 12–13, 14–15, 19, 113
food cravings, 102–3, 130–31
fucose, 83

GABA (gamma-aminobutyric acid), 10–11, 217
galactose, 82–83
garlic, 228
genetics and mental illness, 27–43
  case study, 27–33
  compensation by genes, 34–35
  metal metabolism, 41–42
  methylation, 38–41
  pyroluria (pyrrole disorder), 36, 37

research, 33–34
 violence and, 35–36
Gerber, Richard, 187
Gershon, Michael, 34, 98–99
Giardia lamblia, 141
Giffen, Bruce, 96
Gina (case study), 158–63
Glenmullen, Joseph, 15, 16
glucosamine (N-acetylglucosamine, NAG), 84
glucose, 82
glutamate, 88
glutamic acid, 88–89, 132, 218
glutamine, 88, 217, 218
glutathione, 104, 119
glyconutrients (monosaccharides), 81–85
 case study, 79–80
 fucose, 83
 galactose, 82–83
 glucose, 82
 mannose, 83–84
 N-acetylgalactosamine, 83
 N-acetylglucosamine (NAG, glucosamine), 84
 N-acetylneuraminic acid (NANA), 84
 supplements, 84–85
 xylose, 83
glycoproteins, 81–82
grapeseed extract, 228
Green, Steven (case study), 106–12

Hahnemann, Christian Frederick Samuel, 200–201, 204
Hammond, Corydon, 157

Hands of Light (Brennan), 189
Hartford, Haley (case study), 77–80
Hay, Louise L., 178–79
Healing Visualizations (Epstein), 180
HEG, 156
hemoencephalography (HEG), 156
hippocampus, 165
histamine, 11, 39–40
HLA, 42–43
homeopathy, 196–204
 case study, 196–99
 effectiveness studies, 203
 history of, 200–202
 practitioners, finding, 204
 treatments, 202
 vs. allopathy, 203–4
Hope, Kirsten, 198
hormone replacement therapy, 74
hormones, 60–76
 adrenal, 70
 balancing, 76
 case study, 60–65
 cortisol, 71–72
 DHEA, 70–71
 estrogen, 73–74
 insulin, 71
 melatonin, 72
 progesterone, 74–75
 testosterone, 75
 thyroid, 64–65, 67
Howell, Edward, 100
5-HTP, 86–87, 131
human leukocyte antigen (HLA), 42–43
Hutchison, Michael, 169
hyperthyroidism, 67

hypoglycemia, 71
hypothalamus, 165
hypothyroidism, 67–70

Ibric, Victoria L., 151
IgE (immunoglobulin E), 97–98
imagery, 174–75, 179–80
immune system
    allergies and, 97–98
    celiac disease, 42–43
    digestion and, 99–100
immunoglobulins, 97–98
Impossible Cure (Lansky), 200
inflammation, 28, 223–25
infrared saunas, 120
insect parasites, 142
insulin, 71
iodine, 55, 70
iron, 55–56, 116

Jasper, Cary, 175
Jensen, Mary (case study),
    90–97
Journal of Clinical Psychology, 167
*Journal of the American Academy of
    Child and Adolescent Psychiatry*, 7
*Journal of the American Geriatrics
    Society*, 182
*Journal of the American Medical
    Association*, 68
Joy (case study), 60–65

Khalsa, Dharma, 71, 181
Kirlian, Semyon, 189
Kripke, D. F., 167
Kropp, Tim, 117

Lactobacillus acidophilus, 125
The Lancet, 68, 203
Langley, John, 12
Lansky, Amy L., 200
lead, 114, 119–20
leaky gut, 99, 104
Lee, Lita, 101–2
Lefkowitz, Doris, 83
Leighton, Stephen, 64–65
LENS (Low Energy Neurofeedback
    System), 156
Levinson, Andrew, 109–10
light therapy, 167–69
limbic system, 165
lipase, 100
Lipski, Elizabeth, 125
lithium, 18, 46, 60–65, 122–23
liver, 118–21
Loomis, Howard F., Jr., 101
Ludwig, Hanns, 143

magnesium, 56, 105
magnetic resonance imaging (MRI),
    4
magnets, 63–64
Mahikari no Waza, 92–93
major depression, 5
mania
    diseases or conditions that may
        trigger, 66
    drugs that cause, 67
    symptoms, 6–7
Mannatech supplements, 80, 81, 85
mannose, 83–84
McAnalley, Bill H., 81, 85
McDaniel, H. Reginald, 81

meditation, 181–82
melatonin, 72
mercury
  case study, 106–12
  detoxification, 119–20
  effects of, 113–14
  sources of, 112–13
meridians, 191
metallothionein, 41
metals
  balancing, 106
  case study, 106–12
  detoxification, 118–21
  essential, 115–16
  metabolism of, 41–42
  toxic, 112–15
methadone, 65
methionine, 40, 87, 217, 218
methylation, 38–41
mild depression, 5
mindfulness, 182
minerals and the brain, 54–57
mineral supplements, 216
molybdenum, 56
monoamine oxidase inhibitors
    (MAOIs), 17–18
monosaccharides. *see* glyconutrients
monosodium glutamate (MSG),
    132–34
mood stabilizers, 18
Moore, Neecie, 79, 80
Moses, Marion, 117–18
Mount Sinai School of Medicine,
    117
MRI (magnetic resonance imaging),
    4

MSG, 132–34
Myss, Carolyn, 183

N-acetylgalactosamine, 83
N-acetylglucosamine (NAG,
    glucosamine), 84
N-acetylneuraminic acid (NANA),
    84
Nambudripad, Devi S., 94
Nambudripad's Allergy Elimination
    Techniques (NAET), 94–95, 96
Nasse, John, 46
National Academy of Sciences, 117
National Institute of Mental Health
    (NIMH) Human Genetics
    Initiative, 33–34
National Institutes of Health, 33,
    34, 191
National Mental Health
    Association, 7
Natural Hormone Balance for Women
    (Reiss), 75
naturopaths, 28, 76, 197, 198,
    210–12, 215. *see also*
    homeopathy
NeuroReports, 113–14
nervous system and mood disorders,
    9–11
neurofeedback, 149–57
  case study, 149–52
  depression and brain-wave
    patterns, 157
  history of, 153–54
  treatments, 151, 156–57
  types of brain waves, 154–56
neuroleptic malignant syndrome, 19

neurons, 9, 153
neurotransmitters
    minerals and, 54–57
    mood disorders and, 9–11
    protein and, 81
    vitamins and, 50–54
New England Journal of Medicine, 70
niacin (vitamin B₃), 51
Nicole (case study), 149–52
norepinephrin (noradrenaline), 11
nutrigenomics, 38

O'Connor, Deirdre, 28–29, 42
OHHPL, 37
The Omega-3 Connection (Stoll), 31,
    32, 58, 194
omega-3 fatty acids, 58
omega-6 fatty acids, 58
oregano oil, 228
organic affective syndrome, 110
Othmer, Siegfried, 155–56
overmethylation, 40–41

pantothenic acid (vitamin B₅),
    51–52
parasites, 136–46
    case study, 140–41
    contracting, 144
    prevention, 144–45
    protozoa infection program,
        233–38
    testing for, 146
    types and effects of infection,
        141–43
PCBs (polychlorinated biphenyls),
    117–18

PEA, 87–88, 134–35
pesticides, 117–18
PET, 4
pets, parasites from, 144
Pfeiffer, Carl, 30, 35, 39–40
Pfeiffer Treatment Center, 30–31,
    35–36, 39–40, 41, 42
pharmaceutical industry, 13–14, 16,
    20
phenylalanine, 87–88, 217
phenylethylamine (PEA), 87–88,
    134–35
physical exam/tests, 218
physicians, finding, 214–16
pituitary gland, 165
placebo effect, 183
positron emission tomography
    (PET), 4
postpartum depression, 6, 75
post-traumatic stress disorder
    (PTSD), 164, 166, 167, 169
potassium, 56
potentization, 202
Pottinger, Francis, 101
prana, 188
prayer, 172, 178, 182–83
pregnant and nursing women,
    16
processed foods, 101
Procyk, Anne, 210–12
progesterone, 74–75
protease, 100, 101–2
proteins, 81, 85–86
protozoa infection, 141–42, 233–38.
    see also parasites
Prozac Backlash (Glenmullen), 15

psychiatric drugs, 11–21
    children and, 16
    clinical trials and research, 13–15,
        20
    discontinuing, 21, 214, 219–20
    health risks of, 20
    history of, 11–12
    increasing use of, 11–12
    patient response studies, 13
    prescribing by trial and error, 14
    side effects, 17–21
    withdrawal effects, 219–20
Psychiatric Times, 155–56
PTSD, 164, 166, 167, 169
pyridoxine (vitamin B$_6$), 37, 52
pyroluria (pyrrole disorder), 36, 37

Quiet Mind, 50

Raineau, Lindsae (case study), 184–87
raw foods, 100–101
reflexology, 186–87
reiki, 188, 190, 192–93
Reiss, Uzzi, 75
Renshaw, Perry E., 57
Reston, James, 191
riboflavin (vitamin B$_2$), 51
Rogers, Bonnie, 193
Rosenthal, N. E., 167–68
ROSHI technique, 151, 156
Ross, Julia, 129, 131, 139, 152

SAD, 6, 73, 168, 169
SAMe (S-adenosyl-L-methionine),
    38, 39, 40, 87
saturated fats, 57

Schiffer, Frederick, 168
schizophrenia, 34, 39–40
Schmook, Andrea (case study),
    95–96, 170–77
seasonal affective disorder (SAD), 6,
    73, 168, 169
secondary depression, 6
The Second Brain (Gershon), 34,
    98–99
selective serotonin reuptake
    inhibitors (SSRIs), 11–12,
    15–16, 17
selenium, 56–57
sensorimotor rhythm (SMR), 153,
    154–56
serotonin, 10, 11–12, 15–16, 130
Shannon, Tim, 197, 198
Shapiro, Francine, 165
sleep, 72–73
SMR (sensorimotor rhythm), 153,
    154–56
SSRIs, 11–12, 15–16
Sterman, Barry, 153
Stoll, Andrew, 31, 32, 58, 194
stress
    allergic reactions and, 105
    cortisol and, 71–72
    pyroluria (pyrrole disorder) and,
        37
Strick, Frank, 142
Strogatz, Steve, 72
Sudarshan Kriya Yoga, 181
sugar, 103, 130–31. *see also*
    glyconutrients
    (monosaccharides)
sugar intolerance, 101

sugar substitutes, 131–32
Suzy (case study), 196–99
Sync (Strogatz), 72

tardive akathisia, 19
tardive dyskinesia, 19
tardive dystonia, 19
taurine, 89, 218
T-cells, 42–43
testosterone, 75
thalamus, 165
therapeutic touch, 187–88, 190, 193–95
theta waves, 155
thiamine (vitamin B$_1$), 51
thyroid hormones (tri-iodothyronine [T$_3$], thyroxine [T$_4$]), 64–65, 67–70
tics, 15–16, 18–19
tobacco, 130
tocopherol (vitamin E), 54
Toxoplasma gondii (toxoplasmosis), 142
tranquilizers, 18–19
trans-fatty acids, 59
Treatise on Materia Medica (Cullen), 201
TRH (thyrotropin-releasing hormone), 68
tricyclic antidepressants, 17
tri-iodothyronine (T$_3$). *see* thyroid hormones
trimethylglycine (TMG), 40
Truehope, 31–32, 47, 48, 49
The Truth About the Drug Companies (Angell), 13
tryptophan, 86–87, 217

TSH (thyroid-stimulating hormone), 68
Tulane University School of Medicine, 143
Tylenol PM, 60
tyrosine, 88, 217

undermethylation, 40
University of Calgary Medical School, 113–14
Usui, Mikao, 192–93

Vasquez, Steven, 168, 169
Veltheim, John, 198
Vibrational Medicine (Gerber), 187
Vickie (case study), 136–41
violence, 35–36
viruses, 143
vitamin A, 53
vitamin B$_1$ (thiamine), 51
vitamin B$_2$ (riboflavin), 51
vitamin B$_3$ (niacin), 51
vitamin B$_5$ (pantothenic acid), 51–52
vitamin B$_6$ (pyridoxine), 37, 52
vitamin B$_9$ (folic acid, folate), 41, 52
vitamin B$_{12}$ (cobalamin), 52
vitamin C (ascorbic acid), 53
vitamin D, 53–54
vitamin E (tocopherol), 54
vitamin supplements, 216

Walsh, William, 30, 35–36, 41, 106
Walton, Ralph, 132
Weintraub, Amy, 181, 182
Weintraub, Skye, 132, 133
Wellbutrin, 29, 46

What's a Nice Person Like Me Doing in a Body Like This (Moore), 79
Whitaker, Julian, 127
Wilson, E. Denis, 69
Wilson's thyroid syndrome, 64, 69

xenoestrogens, 74
x-ray computerized tomography (CT), 4
xylose, 83

yeast. *see Candida albicans* (yeast)
Yiamouyiannis, John, 135
yoga, 180–81, 182
Yoga for Depression (Weintraub), 181
You Can Heal Your Life (Hay), 178–79

zinc, 37, 57, 106, 116
Zoloft, 77–78

A Note on the Author

GRACELYN GUYOL is a former public relations executive who was diagnosed with mild bipolar disorder in 1993. Unwilling to remain on antidepressants because of serious side effects, she successfully used drug-free therapies to end her depression and mania several years ago. An informed health advocate, she organizes holistic healing seminars, lectures, and writes about natural health, and has coauthored with members of the Stonington Garden Club a booklet on chemical-free gardening. This is her first book. She lives in Stonington, Connecticut.